KILLED

ON CONTACT

The Tea Tree
Oil Story:
Nature's Finest
Antiseptic

Cass Igram, D.O.

Literary Visions Publishing, Inc.

Literary Visions Publishing, Inc.
Cedar Rapids, Iowa

Printed by Cedar Graphics
P.O. Box 1451
Cedar Rapids, Iowa 52401
For ordering information call
(319) 366-5335

Also by the Same Author

Eat Right to Live Long
Who Needs Headaches?
The Survivor's Nutritional Pharmacy
A Disaster Survival Guide

Printed On Recycled Paper
Made from 100% waste paper fibers

ISBN: 0911119-49-3

printed on
recycled paper

Disclaimer: The contents of this book are not intended as a substitute for medical treatment. Individuals with serious medical illnesses should consult their physicians before beginning new treatments and/or altering existing treatment programs.

Table of Contents

Introduction

In today's age billions of dollars are spent by Americans each year on prescription and over the counter medicines. Unfortunately, most of these medicines are incapable of curing disease. Rather, they function primarily to ameliorate or modify symptoms. This is true for virtually all categories of drugs other than possibly antibiotics and hormones. Nitroglycerin is a classic example. It suppresses the sensations of anginal (cardiac) pain, and this serves the purpose of reducing the patient's suffering and anxiety. Yet, nitroglycerin does nothing to cure heart disease. The mechanism which causes the chest pain remains. The same is true of anti-hypertensive agents. While they effectively repress blood pressure, the pressure will rise to its original levels as soon as the medicine is stopped. A similar situation is seen with mood-altering medications such as Valium, Prozac and Xanax. Their effects are also temporary, and they often serve only to increase the degree of the mental aberrations and deepen the depression. Thus, it is evident that through the use of such medicines, diseases and symptoms are at best controlled and at worst perpetuated. Long-term cures are rarely achieved.

Symptom control may serve valuable purposes. In fact, control may prove life-saving. Such is often the case with the use of insulin to "control" diabetes and theophylline to "control" asthma. Thyroid hormone is useful for controlling hypothyroidism and is, in fact, a cure for this disease. Yet, even in these diseases the use of medicines as the sole treatment usually leads to unsatisfactory results in terms of achieving optimal health.

The American public is interested in the relief of symptoms but is also interested in finding and utilizing cures. To a degree the medical profession is pursuing cures. Billions of dollars are spent each year performing research to find them. Yet, few cures have been discovered by them to date.

The majority of people, whether suffering from acute or chronic disease, are highly motivated to find cures for their conditions in order to get rid of their illnesses once and for all. However, many fail to discover them in their lifetimes and continue to suffer with whatever ailments they might have, resorting to symptom control through drug therapy as the only means of treatment. Yet, there exist numerous curative agents for the majority of diseases. It's just that most people, as well as the majority of doctors and pharmacists, are unaware that such cures exist. People are even less aware that the majority of the cures are found in Nature, not in the PDR. One of the most valuable of these is tea tree oil.

Tea tree oil is a natural substance offering tremendous curative powers. It is a light-colored and light-weight oil extracted from a shrub-like tree found only in Australia. While relatively unknown in America, this oil is found in nearly all of the pharmacies in Australia. There it is used as a front-line treatment for a variety of common complaints ranging from acne to vaginitis.

In the United States tea tree oil is best known as a treatment for fungal infections, specifically fungal infections of the skin. Currently, it is dispensed primarily from health food outlets, although a small percentage of pharmacies carry it.

Wouldn't it be nice to have available an effective and reliable cure for athlete's foot? What about toenail fungus? Ringworm? Jock itch? Vaginitis? Wouldn't it be great to have access a product which would assuredly provide relief for a variety of common ailments with no side effects.

Tea tree oil is most correctly described as a distillate from the leaves and fronds of the Australian tea tree. This tree, which is found only in an isolated portion of New South Wales, Australia, is known botanical as *Melaluca alternifolia*. While the oil is indeed a potent treatment for fungal infections of the skin, it has hundreds of other uses. These include:

*abrasions
*acne
*allergic rashes, including poison ivy, sumac and oak
*athlete's foot
*bed sores
*bee stings
*boils
*bromhidrosis (sweaty feet)
*canker sores
*caries or root infections
*cold sores
*cradle cap
*cuts
*cystitis
*dandruff
*dermatitis
*diaper rash
*ear infections
*eczema
*furunculosis
*genital herpes
*gingivitis
*halitosis
*head lice
*hemorrhoids
*herpes simplex
*hives
*impetigo
*insect bites
*jock itch
*paronychia

*pruritus
*psoriasis
*ringworm
*scabies
*seborrheic dermatitis
*sinusitis
*snake bites
*sore throats
*thrush
*tonsillitis
*vaginitis

This is certainly a wide range of conditions treatable by a single substance. The fact that it could have so many uses seems incredible. Yet, there is an extensive amount of clinical as well as research evidence supporting the use of tea tree oil for these and many other conditions.

Most of the aforementioned conditions are infectious diseases, and this may explain why tea tree oil offers such extensive utility. Tea tree oil is a potent antiseptic.

Americans have a logical mind set for dealing with health problems: they want results. If a product works, if it lives up to its claims, that product will sell on its own volition. There are thousands of bogus products. Because of this, results-producing products stand out like diamonds in the rough. With such products price is not so important as is effectiveness and safety.

Products which cure conditions rather than suppress symptoms are in great demand. Certainly, such products would be excellent additions to any supermarket, pharmacy or health food store. Tea tree oil is one of those unique and versatile products that it should become a household word.

CHAPTER 1   Antiseptic Par Excellence

There is a substance, little known in America, which has special curative powers beyond anything available in the Western pharmacopeia. It is not a drug but is a product of nature. This substance is tea tree oil, a complex oil consisting of over forty-eight different natural compounds. Tea tree oil is distilled from the leaves (and fronds) of the Australian tea tree. It is a completely natural substance and constitutes a unique blend of a variety of active ingredients, some of which have not been found in any other plant.

The complex chemical nature of tea tree oil is one reason that it has never become available in the pharmacies of the Western world. Try as they might, pharmaceutical houses have been unable to produce it. It is and will always be exclusively a product of Nature, one created by a careful process that only Nature could devise.

Even if the active ingredients in this oil were isolated and synthesized, the synthetic product would be inferior in terms of curative powers than the original natural form. Plus, the synthetic compounds would be more toxic.

Nature, the master of synthesis, has produced tea tree oil as a fine balance of many different yet cooperative components. Some of these components are so unique that their chemical formulas have yet to be elucidated. Only a few can be produced synthetically. Researchers tested some of these synthetic compounds and found them far less potent than the unaltered natural oil. Thus, the various compounds found in tea tree oil, whether occurring in trace amounts or as major components, work synergistically to achieve their therapeutic effects. Despite the complexity of its chemical make-up and the wide range of its uses, its primary value is simple: antisepsis.

The discovery of the astounding antiseptic powers of tea tree oil is no surprise to those who have traversed the Australian bush-lands. Tea tree oil is derived from one of Australia's hardiest and most disease resistant trees: *Melaluca alternifolia*.

Tea tree oil is far from a newcomer in the history of antisepsis. It has been utilized to cure infections by the Australian aborigines for thousands of years.

The Western world was first introduced to tea trees when Captain Cook and his crew set foot on Australia in the 18th century. Unaware of its possible medicinal properties they made a tea of its leaves, hence the name "tea tree." Later, settlers began using this favorite Aboriginal remedy for the treatment of various ailments. In particular, they found it invaluable for the treatment and prevention of wound infections.

It was in the 1920's that Arthur Penfold, a foremost Australian chemist, first performed research on this amazing substance. He found proof that tea tree oil did indeed kill germs. In 1925 Penfold determined that the oil was 12 times as potent as phenol, the standard by which all antiseptics were measured at the time.

Penfold went on to conduct extensive clinical trials with medical practitioners over the next six years. His findings were published in 1937, revealing excellent results with the use of tea tree oil in a wide variety of conditions.

Australians began utilizing tea tree oil for treating infected wounds. Pharmacists and doctors began dispensing it as a front-line antiseptic. Bushmen and other adventurers wouldn't enter the wilderness without it. It was standard issue in first aid kits for British and Australian soldiers stationed in the tropics during World War II. This oil was deemed so valuable that workers who processed it were exempt from military service, and demand quickly outstripped supply.

After the war interest in the use of tea tree oil as an antiseptic declined dramatically. So did interest in all natural healing medicines. Penicillin was introduced, and it captured the full attention of the medical profession. This era was dominated by the chemical and, more specifically, pharmaceutical industry. Today, this industry remains the dominant force in medicine. Ever since the production and synthesis of antibiotics, the use of naturally-occurring antiseptics has fallen out of vogue. However, currently there is great interest in less toxic alternatives to the standard antiseptics and antimicrobial agents.

As mentioned, the post-war period was heralded by an explosive growth of a variety of industries specializing in the synthesis of chemicals. In fact, the late 1940's and 50's may be regarded as the *Era of Chemicalization*. Antibiotics quickly captured the interest of medical researchers and practitioners. They were regarded as the cure-all for infectious diseases. Even in Australia the usage of the tea tree oil declined dramatically.

It was not until the 1970's that interest in the product was revived. Then, in the 1970's, Australian companies began researching methods for cultivating the highest therapeutic grade of tea tree. Cultivation of the tea tree proved feasible, making large-scale commercial production of the oil a reality. The Australian producers encouraged researchers to further investigate the oil's value as an antiseptic agent for the treatment of common medical conditions.

Since the 1920's numerous research articles on tea tree oil have appeared in internationally recognized medical journals, including *Obstetrics and Gynecology* and *Medical Journal of Australia*. These articles have delineated the unusually potent antiseptic powers of tea tree oil and have documented its ability to cure a variety of infectious conditions.

The claims for tea tree oil's curative powers may seem exaggerated, yet these effects are very real and are supported by clinical experience and scientific research. It is truly one of the most valuable antiseptics known. As these pages are perused it will become clear that no household or medical pharmacy should be without it.

The fact that essential plant oils can be utilized in the treatment of disease should not come as a surprise to medical professionals. Many non-prescription remedies contain essential oils. For instance, oil of clove and eucalyptus are found in remedies for respiratory diseases. Tea tree oil belongs to the same botanical categorization as these plants: the myrtle family. Clove and eucalyptus oils exhibit specific effects upon the respiratory passages, effects which have been documented scientifically. Tea tree oil is far more versatile that either of these oils. In fact, few if any plant oils can match its tremendous utility.

Some people might recall the "old days" of the pharmacy business which featured antiseptic agents that are now out of vogue. Then, chemicals, such as boric and carbolic acids, were used to kill germs. Carbolic acid, now known as phenol, was the antiseptic of choice. During this period researchers in Australia determined that tea tree oil was twelve times stronger than carbolic acid. Additionally, it was found to be much less toxic to tissues than all other antiseptics tested. These findings provoked further research on the oil's antiseptic properties and on it use in the treatment of various diseases.

Modern Day Antiseptics

The killing of microbes forms the basis of much of modern pharmacology. Thousands of antimicrobial agents currently exist. The categories include antiseptics, germicides, antibiotics and oxidizing agents. Indeed, there has been literally an explosion in the industrial production of these compounds over the last 50 years. The advent of this movement was precipitated by the discovery of penicillin, itself a natural substance, in the 1940's.

There was good reason for this focus. The major cause of fatalities in the first half of this century was not heart disease, cancer, diabetes or any other degenerative disease: it was infectious disease. Doctors found themselves impotent in curbing the death and disability caused by the infectious epidemics of the early 20th Century, epidemics which included tuberculosis, influenza, polio and pneumonia. No wonder the discovery of antimicrobial agents was met with such excitement and optimism. However, it should be remembered that penicillin's discoverer, Alexander Fleming, encountered more skepticism than welcome after his discovery. In fact, like Louis Pasteur, his findings were largely ignored, and it was only after his death that the full potential of his discovery was realized.

To this day microbial infections constitute the prime factor for patient visits to doctors offices and are responsible for more hospitalizations than any other cause. Conditions such as colds, flu, pneumonia, sore throats, vaginitis, cystitis and ear infections dominate visits to doctors offices. Many of these infections are curable through the use of modern antimicrobial agents. However, many others, such as certain viral infections, are not. For instance, no drug is available for curing the common cold.

What is most astounding is that, despite the advent of modern antimicrobial drugs and chemical antiseptics, the incidence of infectious disease is actually on the rise. Epidemics of colds and flu occur every year and, in some instances, several times yearly. Children are besieged with colds, flu, sore throats and ear aches. Adolescents are plagued with colds and flu and are pestered with an annoying and disfiguring infectious condition: acne. Adults suffer with the same ailments in addition to a variety of other infectious diseases. These include bronchitis, infectious arthritis, cystitis, kidney infections, urethritis, venereal diseases and chronic fatigue syndrome, a condition thought to be caused by viral infection. Then there are the fungal infections which are also exceedingly common. They include athlete's foot, jock itch, vaginitis, toenail fungus, fingernail fungus, ringworm and fungal lung infections. The technology which has synthesized sophisticated drugs, such as tetracyclines, penicillins, cephalosporins, sulfa drugs, aminoglycosides and antifungal agents, has been incapable of producing an agent which prevents infections and which can curb the rising tide of infectious diseases in this country.

What's more, microbes are adapting to synthetic chemicals. As a result there now exists a virtual epidemic of infections caused by drug-resistant forms of microbes. Additionally, many viruses are immune to antiseptics, and all are immune to antibiotics. The fact is the virulence of certain viruses is enhanced by antibiotics. This is what happens when mononucleosis is inadvertently treated with ampicillin.

Drug-Resistant Microbes: The Modern Plague?

Hospitals have become breeding grounds for the development of antibiotic-resistant microorganisms. *Nosocomial infections*, that is infections contracted while in the hospital, are the plague of these institutions, and hundreds of patients are affected every year. These infections are the primary cause of hospital fatalities, the elderly and those with depressed immunity being most vulnerable. However, the resistant organisms are so potent that they can infect relatively healthy individuals and rapidly cause serious illness. The contact can be minimal such as breathing hospital air or shaking hands with a carrier. However the more frequent cause is direct contact such as contamination with human secretions or excrement. The importance of human hands as the medium for spreading infectious disease in the hospital setting cannot be over emphasized. Hands become contaminated with saliva, blood, respiratory secretions and excrement, all of which act as media for the spread of infection.

Antibiotic-resistant microbes are highly pathogenic. They aggressively invade human tissues and, in individuals with compromised immunity, may cause potentially fatal infections. The problem is that the battle is fought on a lone front by the immune system, since these organisms are resistant to the majority of drugs. A healthy immune system can usually fight off infection, even by the most pathogenic, drug resistant organisms. However, even healthy individuals can have their health decimated by these organisms.

The salmonella outbreaks which kill and injure thousands every year are caused primarily by antibiotic-resistant strains. So are most outbreaks of staph and strep infections.

Bacteria are masters at genetic engineering. They efficiently splice new DNA and RNA in attempt to alter their structure and/or metabolism. When undergoing stress they mutate, changing their size, form and shape. This is done to avoid death or, more specifically, extinction. Bacteria have a tremendous capacity to evade efforts to exterminate them. In short, bacteria, or, for that matter, any other types of microbes will do everything possible to survive.

Extinction is a reality for mammals, fish, reptiles and birds. However, this is not so with microbes. They will survive despite man's efforts to eradicate them. Even the most "nuclear" attempts to destroy them will meet with failure. Tests by the government proved that microbes were one of the few creatures able to survive nuclear blasts. They were in existence on this planet billions of years before the advent of man and will remain long after man is gone.

No antiseptic or antibiotic has been created with the explicit purpose of extinguishing microbes from the face of the earth. Rather, the objective is to kill them selectively in order to cure and/or prevent diseases.

It is well known that microbes may be found on virtually every object whether animate or inanimate. Attempts have been made to sterilize regions or devices which could serve as sites for the spread of germs. These include various surfaces, for instance, counter-tops, sinks, toilet seats, and floors, or devices such as medical instruments.

Surgical suites receive the greatest scrutiny in the process of sterilization. Every attempt possible is made to ensure a microbe-free environment. However, complete sterility is impossible: the air cannot be sterilized, nor can the various fixtures within a surgical suite. Neither can human skin be sterilized, although the bacterial count on the it can be reduced significantly. That is effectively accomplished by pre-surgical scrubbing.

Great pains are taken by the surgical scrub team to sterilize the skin of patients, particularly skin directly over the operative site. Iodine is the primary antiseptic used, and it is a relatively safe one. Yet, severe allergic reactions to iodine may occur.

If surgeons began using tea tree oil, they could enhance the process of antisepsis many-fold. As a result of its use surgeons would notice a significant reduction in post-operative infections. Additionally, infections of the incision would be reduced to nil, particularly if tea tree oil were applied over the incision after closure.

Many microbes have developed resistance to the commonly used disinfectants. Despite this, antisepsis has greatly reduced surgical morbidity and mortality. At the turn of the century surgical mortality exceeded 50%. Careful hand washing was the first procedure which improved the statistics, and this alone led to a great reduction in the death rate.

Today, infection remains a common cause of post-surgical morbidity and mortality. In fact, it is the number one cause of mortality in all categories of surgery, with gastrointestinal surgery surpassing all others.

Can the current state of antisepsis be improved? Can

post-surgical mortality be reduced?   If improvement is to occur, the answer will assuredly be found in Nature's infinitely rich pharmacopeia rather than from a dramatic breakthrough in synthesis.   In Nature thousands of agents exist which kill microbes while preventing the development of resistance. Let us not forget that penicillin and sulfa drugs were originally natural extracts.

Nature's antiseptics offer the following advantages over their synthetic counterparts:

1. They are relatively non-toxic.

2. It is difficult, if not impossible, for microbes to develop resistance to them.   This is largely a consequence of the complexity of their chemical structure.   Most synthetic antibiotics are single components with relatively simple structures, ones which microbes can "learn" to resist.

3. Many natural antiseptics kill microbes on contact and also inhibit microbial growth for hours or even days after application.   With many synthetic antiseptics the initial microbial kill is followed by the growth of resistant microbes so that several applications must be made to maintain sterility.

Tea Tree Oil: Nature's Antiseptic Par Excellence

Tea tree oil is a completely natural substance which meets all of the aforementioned criteria. It is an invaluable antiseptic, being one of the most diverse antimicrobial agents known.

Numerous scientific studies have been performed concerning the precise antimicrobial powers of tea tree oil. Research in this field began in the 1920's, when an Australian government chemist, Arthur Penfold, began studying the oil. Penfold quickly recognized that tea tree oil had valuable antiseptic powers and that it was a more potent antiseptic than any chemical then known.

In the early 1900's carbolic acid, which is now known as phenol, was the standard antiseptic agent. Penfold found that tea tree oil easily out performed this compound; he determined that it was over 12 times stronger than carbolic acid while being much less toxic to human tissues. It exhibited unusually potent antifungal activity, more so than any other antiseptic used at that time.

Researchers found that a diluted solution of tea tree oil was three to five times more potent than most household disinfectants. Studies performed in the last decade have further elucidated these powers. It has passed the Kelsey-Sykes and the Australian Therapeutic Goods Act tests, the most rigorous antiseptic tests known.

Tea tree oil is highly effective at killing pathogens, even in dilute amounts. A one in fourty dilution killed antibiotic-resistant staph, which are notoriously hard to kill. Tests showed that its microbial killing powers surpassed those of alcohol, and it was nearly as effective as chlorine. Astoundingly, tea tree oil is capable of killing some pathogens in dilutions as weak as 1 in 1000.

Hemolytic streptococci were inhibited in dilutions of 1 in 50, and, amazingly, growth continued to be inhibited for weeks. Studies by E. H. Holland of Australia University in Sydney, Australia, documented tea tree oil's ability to virtually sterilize dilutions of fecal matter. Nearly 50% of the organisms were killed in light dilutions of 1 in 200, and stronger solutions resulted in near complete sterilization. Tea tree oil possesses the unique capacity to penetrate organic matter, which occurs in large amounts in feces; that penetration greatly facilitates its antimicrobial capacity.

Pus-laden fluid, such as that found in infected wounds, is high in organic matter as is blood. Tea tree oil exerts potent antibiotic-like activity within these fluids. It penetrates the organic matter completely helping to sterilize infected wounds. What a valuable antiseptic it is that can sterilize blood and pus.

Tea tree oil is probably best known for its ability to kill fungi. It possesses "unbelievable" fungicidal capacity and can cause complete inhibition of growth in test tubes for up to one month. Other test have documented tremendous activity against bacteria, parasites and viruses.

Organisms against which tea tree oil has been shown to be effective include:

*aspergillus
*bacteroides
*Candida
*clostridium
*cryptosporidium
*diptheroids
*E. Coli
*enterobacter
*epidermophyton
*fusobacterium
*gonococcus
*hemophilus
*herpes viruses
*meningococcus
*microsporium
*peptococcus
*proteus
*pseudomonas
*spirochetes
*staph
*strep
*trichinosis
*trichophyton

Toxicity of Essential Oils

Prior to the advent of antibiotics various chemical antiseptics, such as boric, acetic and carbolic acids, were used as the primary armamentarium against microbes. Too, potassium iodide was dispensed, as was merthiolate. While these agents were being used in the USA, in Australia tea tree oil was the antiseptic of choice. Australians found it to be far more potent than traditional antiseptics and much less irritating to the tissues as well.

In 1930, the *Medical Journal of Australia* featured an article entitled, "A New Australia Germicide." It reported that tea tree oil was effective in curing a variety of conditions, including septic wounds. In fact, localized tissue infections of all types were found to respond, and the benefits included sterilization of the wound, decreased complications and increased rate of healing. Said the Journal, "The results obtained in a variety of conditions...were most encouraging, a striking feature being that it (tea tree oil) dissolved pus and left surfaces of infected wounds clean so that its germicidal action became more effective without any apparent damage to the tissues." This was a new concept in the field of antisepsis, since many of the original germicides destroyed tissue as well as microbes. Indeed, it has been known for decades that common antiseptics, including merthiolate, iodine, hexachlorophene and hydrogen peroxide, cause cellular toxicity and death. The latter two are suspected carcinogens; thus, their usage externally is limited to only the most superficial wounds. Tea tree oil is unique when contrasted to these antiseptics: while just as effective, it causes minimal or no ill effects upon human tissues.

Concerns for toxicity should not be taken lightly. Any agent used in the treatment of disease should be evaluated for potential ill-effects. All chemicals, whether synthetic or natural, are potentially toxic. Even water, which is itself a chemical, can be toxic if consumed in excessive amounts.

Chemicals with potentially greater toxicity, such as medicines, should be carefully scrutinized before being freely prescribed.

It should be emphasized that tea tree oil is an antiseptic. Like all other antiseptics its usage should be limited to external application. Internal consumption should be avoided. Just as one would not be advised to drink iodine, hydrogen peroxide or hexachlorophene, neither is it advisable to consume tea tree oil.

This is not to suggest that tea tree oil is exceptionally toxic when taken internally. There are no deaths on record from internal use or accidental overdose. However, the oil has only been proven safe for external usage. While tea tree oil cannot be regarded as being highly toxic, evidence exists that consumption may lead to internal organ damage. However, the LD 50, the standard method used to measure fatal toxicity, exceeds 30 milliliters. That means that 30 milliliters per day proved fatal to test animals. Small amounts, as in those that might be absorbed as a result of external applications, are non-toxic. Further evidence for its low toxicity is found in the fact that tea tree oil is used as a carrier for natural flavors: for instance, nutmeg oil.

Symptoms resulting from acute poisoning (one ounce or more) include nausea, diaphoresis, confusion, seizures, respiratory depression and coma. Liver enzyme and creatinine levels may be elevated. In the event of accidental ingestion of large amounts, drink copious quantities of water. Do not induce vomiting. Activated charcoal may be of value in absorbing the excess oil if taken promptly.

Tea tree oil finds its greatest usage as a remedial agent for diseases affecting the exposed surfaces and the mucous membranes. It can be safely used in small doses on all mucous membranes, including the gums, oral mucosa, vagina, urethra, colon and rectum. Although internal ingestion has been attempted without noticeable toxic effects, this is not enough evidence to warrant its widespread use internally. In short, until evidence proves otherwise, tea tree oil should be used only for external applications and should not be swallowed. Like other essential oils, it can be used to coat and soothe the inflamed tissues of sore throats and swollen tonsils. Five drops of tea tree oil in 8 ounces of water makes an excellent gargle. It can be inhaled to help relieve bronchial congestion and to aid in opening clogged sinus passages.

Eucalyptus oil is used for the purpose of healing the respiratory passages, and the amount that actually enters the tissues is minimal. It is not advisable to drink eucalyptus oil by the ounce. The same caution should be exercised regarding tea tree oil.

Numerous essential oils have been utilized in the health and beauty industries. Essential oils are defined as naturally-occurring oils extracted from various plants. These oils are composed of a variety of different substances each with their own chemical structures.

In tiny amounts, essential oils are harmless. The potential toxicity from internal consumption is enhanced if the oils are chemically altered or refined. However, some oils are toxic to the skin or mucous membranes if used repeatedly. For instance, certain compounds in lemon and orange oils have been determined to be carcinogenic. Tea tree oil exhibits none of this toxicity to human skin, even if used over prolonged periods. It is one of the least irritating of all essential oils, and allergic reactions to it are uncommon. What's more, the oil is exceptionally safe to use on the delicate mucous membranes. In fact, it soothes these membranes when they are inflamed. Its deep penetrating action helps curb inflammation while leaving no oily residue.

CHAPTER 2

Medical Uses

The medical uses for tea tree oil are vast. This utility can best be comprehended by comparing it with other antiseptics.

Iodine, merthiolate and hydrogen peroxide are common antiseptics found in every pharmacy and in many medicine cabinets. Currently, their usage is limited to topical applications, primarily for wounds. Earlier in this century doctors used iodine to paint the throat and the vaginal tract in order to treat localized infections of these regions. Hydrogen peroxide sees limited use as an antiseptic. It is contraindicated for deep wounds, as it is caustic to the tissues. Merthiolate, which contains mercury, is also contraindicated for deep wounds. In summary, these antiseptics are prescribed almost exclusively for use on minor cuts or wounds. The same is true of Bactine and similar over-the-counter antiseptics.

Antibiotics also have limited applications for topical usage. Currently, they are prescribed for a variety of illnesses of the skin and mucous membranes in attempt to cure or prevent localized infections. The problem is that these antibiotics kill only certain types of microorganisms. Thus, to utilize them optimally it would be necessary to know precisely which organism(s) is/are sensitive to a given drug. It is virtually impossible to routinely perform culture and sensitivity before treating localized infections of the skin and/or mucous membranes. Additionally, in many skin conditions, the causative organism cannot be readily determined through standard laboratory cultures. Plus, there are often numerous causative organisms.

Often, it is impossible to determine even which category of organisms is primarily responsible: viruses, bacteria, yeasts, fungi or parasites. For example, acne is believed to be caused by certain bacteria, which invade the pores, ducts and follicles of the skin. Topical antibacterial agents, such as erythromycins, have been used successfully for acne. However, they fail to cure this distressing disorder. Often, the antibiotics must be taken daily for many months or years in order to keep the acne at bay, a circumstance which inevitably results in toxicity. Vaginitis is caused by a variety of microbes. Thus, most antibiotics are an inappropriate treatment for this condition. Antifungal creams, such as Lotrimin and Mycolog, are useful in the treatment of vaginitis caused by Candida albicans. However, they are useless for the treatment of bacterial, viral or parasitic vaginitis. Topical antibiotics might be an acceptable treatment for uncomplicated or minor wound infections. However, they are inadequate for the treatment of wound infections caused by antibiotic-resistant microbes, as would be seen in hospitalized patients.

This only further emphasizes how incredibly useful tea tree oil is for the treatment of infectious diseases. In contrast to drugs, tea tree oil can be used as the primary treatment for each of the mentioned conditions. In many instances it proves more effective than the medical treatment(s) of choice. This emphasizes an important point: tea tree oil cannot be thought of as a drug which has action against specific microbes only. Rather, it must be looked upon as a universal antiseptic, one capable of curing virtually all types of infections, even those caused by the most stubborn, drug-resistant microbes known. It is only through this bend of mind that the full potential of tea tree oil in the treatment of human disease can be realized. There is nothing incredible about these statements. These are simply the plain facts about this incredibly useful and amazingly effective oil from the swamps of Australia.

Medical professionals will be skeptical about these claims. Many will outright refuse to investigate tea tree oil and/or recommend its use. Yet, only a fool would fail to try it, to experiment with it, to test it; in short, to see first hand if it really works. Doctors are in the perfect position to do so. They have the patients; all they need to do is order a sample of the oil and evaluate precisely what it is capable of doing. This experimentation is the scientific method that medical professionals have been applying for centuries. Pharmacists can also experiment with it. They may order a sample of the oil and use it to treat family members or themselves for some stubborn condition which has failed to respond to their remedies. That is the best way to evaluate tea tree oil.

Clinical results are also important. Let's review some of conditions for which it has been used.

Acne

Acne is a stubborn condition afflicting primarily adolescents and teenagers. It is caused in part by infection of the sebaceous glands, which are found in great numbers on the face, chest and upper back.

Many treatments have been advanced for acne. They include local antiseptics, facial scrubs, oxidizing agents and systemic antibiotics. One of the most effective and best studied treatments is the oxidizing agent *benzyl peroxide*. A recent study performed by Alvin Schemis, M.D., compared the effectiveness of tea tree oil versus benzyl peroxide in the treatment of acne in teenagers. It was found that a minimal concentration of tea tree oil, while taking longer to show positive effects, was equally effective in minimizing the lesions. What's more, it was determined that tea tree oil was less toxic to the sensitive adolescent skin. Benzyl peroxide kills microbes, but it also oxidizes human cells. Tea tree oil kills microbes but does so without damaging skin cells and is particularly valuable treatment for those with sensitive skin who "react to everything."

While not a cure in itself, tea tree oil nearly matched the efficacy of the front line medical treatment for acne. However, the study could be faulted in one respect: not enough tea tree oil was used, and it was not used often enough. It is likely that if a higher concentration of the oil had been applied three times daily greater improvement would have been seen.

Bed Sores and Other Skin Ulcerations

Bed sores are a distressing condition and are rising in incidence dramatically. Bed sores afflict primarily the elderly and infirm. These sores are notorious for failing to heal and for easily becoming infected. They are common in individuals who are bedridden, for instance residents of nursing homes and hospitalized patients.

Varicose ulcers, also known as stasis ulcers, are similar to bed sores in appearance. They are due primarily to stasis of blood flow as a result of poor venous return. People with a history of varicose veins are vulnerable to their development as are diabetics and individuals with atherosclerosis. The latter groups are also vulnerable to ulcerations due to impaired arterial blood flow. Diabetic foot ulcers are an example.

Diabetics frequently develop ulcerations in the extremities, particularly the legs and feet. These ulcers may precede the development of gangrene. The concern of most medical professionals is that the ulcers will become infected. These infections are particularly likely to develop in diabetics or in other individuals who have impaired circulation. Additionally, diabetics suffer from compromised immune function and delayed wound healing. Thus, they are profoundly susceptible to the development of severe wound infections.

Poor circulation impairs the delivery of oxygen and nutrients to the affected region. As a result infection readily develops. Add to this weakened immunity and the infection can quickly spread and, therefore, become serious.

That is why such great care is taken in medical institutions to cleanse open sores and wounds when they develop in the chronically ill. Surgeons frequently cleanse and debride them on a daily basis, and, in some instances, several times each day. The usual focus is on preventing bacterial infection. Local antiseptics, as well as systemic antibiotics, are often prescribed. However, what is less commonly understood is that these lesions are frequently infected by various fungal organisms, and antibiotics do nothing to kill fungi. Rather, they encourage their growth. That is why yeasts are frequently cultured from these wounds, although they are usually regarded as a source of "secondary infection."

It is important to note that fungi grow best upon diseased and/or dead tissue. In a forest one does not see molds and mushrooms growing on healthy trees. They grow prolifically on diseased, dying or dead trees. The same applies to human tissues. Healthy tissues will not allow the growth of invasive fungi.

Tea tree oil is the agent of choice for the topical treatment of bed sores, varicose ulcers and diabetic ulcers. This is because it exhibits both antibacterial and antifungal activity. It is ideal for use on open wounds, since it penetrates deep into the injured tissue and coats both healthy and diseased portions. It helps sterilize the wound and its secretions. It disperses pus. It prevents the development of further infections by opportunistic organisms. Plus, it helps speed the healing of these difficult to cure wounds.

Tea tree oil should be used as a front line treatment on all types of open wounds seen in bedridden and debilitated patients. These wounds include post-surgical wounds, bed sores, varicose ulcers, diabetic ulcers, ulcers due to impaired arterial flow and gangrenous lesions. Even if other measures are prescribed, tea tree oil should be used as an adjunctive therapy. It should routinely be applied on open wounds which are being treated through the use of systemic antibiotics. This is so that localized as well as systemic fungal overgrowth may be prevented. As such, it should be made readily available for dispensing in hospitals and pharmacies.

The tremendous value of tea tree oil in the treatment of these lesions lies to a large degree in its potent action against fungi. Fungi are parasites; in other words, they are opportunists. They invade weakened and diseased tissues. They are unable to invade healthy tissue.

Once fungi parasitize the tissues, they are difficult to eradicate. Thus, in the case of bed sores the immune system is faced with the burden of eliminating both the initial bacterial infection and the secondary fungal infection. Tea tree oil helps remove that added burden from the immune system, allowing more efficient eradication of bacterial infections. The result is that the wounds will heal more quickly and completely.

Physicians know that if stubborn infections develop in open wounds or other injured tissues, complications are likely. This is particularly true of the elderly and those with compromised immunity. The high mortality rate from hip fractures in the elderly is not due to the fractures themselves; it is due to the complications arising afterward, one of which is infection. The same is true of diabetes and cancer. Opportunistic infections are responsible for a greater number of deaths in cancer victims than any other factor.

The key to curing open sores is to quickly eradicate the infection and prevent further infections from developing. If this is accomplished the rate of healing can be expected to double or even triple.

Tea tree oil exerts potent antimicrobial action on or within human tissues. In fact, its antiseptic powers are enhanced in tissue when compared to the test tube. It penetrates deep into the wound, saturating and coating damaged tissues. It permeates pus, helping to break-up pockets of infection and helps prevent secretions from spreading and maintaining the infection. It destroys fungi on contact, kills most bacteria and inhibits the growth of virtually all other opportunistic microbes.

In the chronically ill, skin ulcerations must be regarded seriously. In diabetics, open wounds may proceed to more serious conditions: gangrene and amputation. If the infection can be rapidly eliminated, the wound will heal by secondary intention and the crisis will be resolved. Infected wounds which are treated with tea tree oil can be sterilized within minutes. Hence, this oil can help save both limbs and lives.

Boils

There are two types of boils: carbuncles and furuncles. The distinction is that carbuncles are infections within the sebaceous glands of the skin while furuncles are infections within the hair follicles. This latter condition commonly occurs in men with heavy beards who shave frequently. Shaving causes micro-trauma to the delicate facial skin and microbes may gain entrance to the hair follicles through tiny cracks in the skin.

Black males are particularly susceptible, as they may develop a unique type of furunculosis due to ingrown hairs on the face and other regions. These boils often occur in large numbers on the cheeks and/or neck.

Most furuncles and carbuncles are caused by staph and/or strep infections. However, infection by yeasts may be a contributing cause.

While boils are often painful and/or disfiguring, they are not regarded as a serious condition. However, if left untreated they may persist for weeks or months. Systemic antibiotic therapy usually provides disappointing results. This is due to the fact that it is difficult to deliver enough of the drug to the site of the infection. Plus, the infections are often caused by antibiotic-resistant microbes, staphylococcus being one of the most notorious of these. People who co-exist in close quarters, such as athletic teams or hospital patients, may suffer from outbreaks of staphylococcal boils.

Often, janitorial workers attempt to sterilize surfaces and fixtures in order to stop the outbreaks. This frequently meets with failure and the infections continue to recur. The addition of tea tree oil to the sterilization mixture would greatly improve the results. The oil could also be added to the wash cycle to aid in the destruction of pathogens that reside on uniforms and other clothing. In gymnasiums, benches, floors, wrestling mats and various fixtures could be washed with a tea tree oil soap solution. Staph which are resistant to standard antiseptics would quickly be destroyed if tea tree oil were added to the sterilizing solution.

Excision and drainage may provide relief, but it is likely that the boils will recur. Thus, surgery is regarded as the last resort in treatment. The use of local antiseptics is the most logical approach and is also the least traumatic. In a recent study it was found that of 25 cases of patients with recurring boils, 24 were cured through the use of tea tree oil without the need for excision. In the control group one-half required excision and drainage.

Tea tree oil is most effective if applied immediately after the boil develops. If the individual has a propensity for the occurrence of boils in certain regions, diluted tea tree oil can be massaged into the skin or mucous membranes preventively. Of note, a dilute solution of tea tree oil in warm water makes an excellent after shave tonic.

Surgical excision, if performed repeatedly, is likely to result in disfiguring scars. With the regular use of tea tree oil, boils can be cured and/or prevented and scars will be entirely avoided.

Bromhidrosis

Bromhidrosis, or sweaty feet, is a condition which commonly afflicts Americans. It is more specifically defined as sweating of the feet without exercise. The condition occurs in children, teenagers and adults. It is often attributed to nervousness.

The most unsettling aspect of bromhidrosis is that the sweaty feet are usually malodorous. When the feet sweat the added moisture increases the likelihood for microbial overgrowth, since moisture encourages the growth of microbes, particularly yeasts. The most vulnerable site for this is between the toes, the region where moisture is most easily retained. To treat this condition apply tea tree oil liberally over the soles of the feet and between the toes twice daily. Continue applications until the odor diminishes, and then apply once daily as a maintenance.

Burns

It may seem astonishing that such a potent germicide could be used safely on highly sensitive and delicate tissues such as those seen in burns. Medical experts are cautious in respect to what compounds they apply on burned tissues and rightfully so. The problem is that more damage may be done than with no treatment, since most antiseptics are caustic. In contrast, tea tree oil is non-toxic to burned tissue. When applied to burns it tends to deaden the pain. It's anesthetic-like action is so soothing that it often gives immediate relief to burn victims.

Researchers at the Australian Health Department's Royal North Shore Hospital in Sydney have determined that regular applications of tea tree oil entirely prevented the development of infections in 1st and 2nd degree burns. The most recent findings indicate that the oil accelerates the healing of deep and superficial skin layers while preventing scarring. That makes it invaluable for the treatment of burns both in the field and in the hospital setting.

Infection commonly develops as a complication of severe burns. Second and third degree burns nearly always become infected if no treatment is applied. Daily administration of tea tree oil on the burn sites will prevent infection of the skin and subcutaneous tissues even in the most severe of burns.

Diaper Rash

This common condition of infants is not simply a rash; it is an infection of the skin usually caused by yeasts. The primary culprit is Candida albicans. Application of diluted tea tree oil, such as a 5% in a cream, results in clearance of the lesions and immediate relief of discomfort in the majority of cases. For optimal results the diluted oil or cream should be applied morning and night after careful washing. Avoid using harsh soaps, as they could cause further irritation. Care must be taken to ensure adequate hygiene, since excrement acts as a carrier for the yeasts.

The baby may be a carrier for yeasts and may suffer from vaginal and/or intestinal overgrowth. As a result oral drugs, such as Nystatin, may need to be prescribed in addition to topical treatment. Taking acidophilus supplements plus the ingestion of yogurt would be a preferable approach and may prove equally as effective as Nystatin in clearing the internal infection. Acidophilus bacteria and other normal flora inhibit the growth of yeasts.

If the mother is breast feeding, she too may require treatment with antifungal agents and/or acidophilus cultures. Breast-feeding mothers should avoid consuming drugs whenever possible, since these chemicals will be transferred into the breast milk and passed on to the baby. Breast milk is of the mother and whatever she eats, drinks and whatever medicine she takes will be in it.

Researchers have determined that yogurt contains a variety of friendly bacteria primarily of the lactobacillus species. The human body naturally contains billions of these bacteria. However, billions of potentially pathogenic microbes also live within it. The key is balance, and the element that maintains this balance is the friendly bacteria.

Once the friendly bacteria are ingested, they populate the mucous membranes of the gut. Additionally, they may be absorbed into the bloodstream. From here they are concentrated into breast milk. Noxious microbes may also be transported from the bowel into the blood and end up in the milk. These facts emphasize the importance of treating both the mother and the infant in preventing Candida overgrowth.

Tea tree oil, preferably in cream or ointment form, can be swabbed on the inflamed skin of diaper rash and can also be applied about the anus and genitals. Even the most stubborn cases of diaper rash will respond to this treatment, and results are usually seen within 24 hours.

Babies with ultra-sensitive skin may not tolerate tea tree oil at full strength. In such instances use tea tree oil lotions or creams. If none of these are available apply a dilute solution (1 in 10) of tea tree oil in olive oil. If the rash or inflammation worsens or fails to respond, consult your physician immediately.

Ear Infections

Ear infections are one of the most common infectious diseases of modern times. The incidence of this condition has risen dramatically over the last 50 years. In particular, ear infections plague infants and children. Adults rarely develop them.

For parents ear aches are among the most frightening of the infectious conditions suffered by their children. There are several reasons for the parents' worries. They know how painful ear aches are and, thus, are concerned about the degree of suffering that their children experience. There is also the concern about the possibility that ear infections could spread to other parts of the body, notably the brain. This is what scares parents the most about these infections.

It is true that the inner and middle ear cavities are in close proximity to the brain. Infection of the brain in children is relatively rare, but when it occurs it is frequently fatal. These infections include meningitis, encephalitis and brain abscess.

The truth is these fears are exaggerated. An incredibly small percentage of cases of ear infections lead to brain or spinal cord infection. The vast majority of cases of meningitis, encephalitis or brain abscesses are caused as a consequence of other factors. Some of these include poor hygiene, blood poisoning, animal bites, insect bites, pneumonia and surgery (and its complications). People should be equally concerned about these factors as they are about ear infections.

The current approach in medicine is to aggressively treat ear infections with prescription medicines. Frequently, when treating this condition, doctors prescribe dose after dose of potent drugs like broad-spectrum antibiotics, cortisone and codeine.

Pediatricians are notorious for prescribing antibiotics for virtually all childhood illness. Children, particularly infants, are easily overdosed by such medicines and numerous side effects may result. Antibiotics are far from innocuous. Occasionally, the ill effects from these drugs proves life-threatening.

A variety of illnesses can be induced as a consequence of prolonged antibiotic therapy. They include chronic candidiasis, chronic serous otitis media, irritable bowel syndrome, pseudomembranous colitis and food intolerance.

While it is true that the appropriate treatment of severe ear infections may include the use of prescription antibiotics either as oral doses or ear drops, rarely, if ever, is the use of codeine indicated. Codeine and all other opiates are nervous system depressants. Thus, they depress the function of all organ systems, which are ultimately controlled by the nervous system. Its ill effects upon respiration are of particular concern. If lung function is depressed less oxygen will be available for the tissues and the results may be catastrophic. Impaired function of the immune system will result, and the function of the brain, our body's number one oxygen consumer, may be seriously impaired. If this respiratory depression occurs a prolonged period, seizures and/or coma may result. Additionally, the systemic physiological depression induced by codeine increases the tendency for infections to spread. As a result a self-limiting disease can be turned into a fatal one.

Today, medical authorities disagree on the potential value of long-term antibiotic therapy for the treatment and/or prevention of ear infections. Nearly all agree that youngsters are at risk of significant side-effects when such medicines are used over lengthy periods.

The prolonged use of antibiotics causes the destruction of most of the bacteria in the bowel, and the friendly bacteria are hit particularly hard. They are less able to develop resistance to antibiotics than are the pathogens. The destruction of the friendly bacteria creates a void, and the result is that the growth of pathogenic organisms is encouraged. The growth of yeasts is also greatly accelerated as a consequence of destruction of the normal flora, since the latter secrete a variety of substances which inhibit the growth of fungi. Some researchers have discovered that with children prolonged antibiotic therapy may itself cause a type of chronic otitis media: that due to Candida albicans.

Antibiotics negatively affect immunity. Most antibiotics impair white blood cell function. Evidence exists that they cause a significant reduction in the *phagocytic index*, a measurement of the ability of white blood cells to destroy microbes. The reduction in immune potential encourages the development of opportunistic infections, the very thing that doctors are attempting to cure.

Medical professionals are aware that long-term use of potent medicines increases patients' risks for developing a variety of ailments. Infants and children are significantly more vulnerable to these ill effects than are adults.

Medicines can become addictive, and this is particularly

true of mood-altering drugs such as the opiates. Codeine should be prescribed with great caution in children, and its use should be prohibited in infants. Drug dependency to codeine is relatively common in America. This problem is due in part to the ease of availability of codeine in prescription medications. Medical professionals should do everything possible to avoid encouraging opiate dependency and limiting the prescription of codeine in the pre-adult population would prove helpful in this regard.

Ear drops are another common treatment for ear aches and are utilized to treat both middle and outer ear infections. Often, with outer ear infections no other treatment is required. The active ingredients in these drops vary from antibiotics to cortisone and acetic acid.

Tea tree oil should not be dripped into the ear. It is safe to use on the outer ear. For the treatment of outer ear infections soak a cotton ball with tea tree oil and hold it against the ear orifice. To reiterate, only prescription drugs should be dripped into the ear canal. Fortunately, tea tree oil is well absorbed into the ear canal through this indirect contact, and this treatment alone will help reduce the pain and inflammation in most instances. The same "indirect" approach can be used for the treatment of middle ear infections.

Tea tree oil is a useful adjunct in the standard treatment for ear infections. It may be used in conjunction with oral antibiotics. Relief is rapid, and infants respond the quickest. In the usual case, improvement is seen within 24 hours. Mothers may notice that the infants become less irritable and that crying spells, fever and pulling at the ear lessen. As the infection is cleared, fever and chills dissipate.

There is a word of caution: as always, consult your physician if and when your child/children become ill. Tea tree oil is simply a supportive therapy useful for enhancing the therapies prescribed by your physician. Do not attempt to treat this condition on your own.

Outer Ear Infections

Swimmer's ear is a common type of outer ear infection. It afflicts mainly children and teenagers. It occurs almost exclusively during the summer months.

Water in swimming pools, lakes or seas may become contaminated with pathogens. When the levels of these pathogens in natural waters reaches certain levels, swimming is banned. However, even during "legal" swimming periods, a large enough number of these organisms remain in the water to cause human diseases. These water-borne pathogens readily infect the outer ear canal. They include viruses, bacteria, bacteria-like organisms, fungi, protozoans, amebas and parasitic worms.

The vast majority of outer ear infections are caused by bacteria and fungi. The skin of the outer ear offers a moist, nutrient-rich environment, which is precisely what these organism require for their growth. Candida commonly infects the outer ear canal, and long term usage of antibiotics and/or birth control pills increases the likelihood for the development of this infection. Symptoms depend upon whether the infection is acute or chronic. In acute infection symptoms include pain, aching and discharge. With chronic infection the symptoms are primarily fullness in the ear, excessive wax, irritation and itching.

To treat this condition simply place one drop of the oil directly onto the outer ear region morning and night. To repeat, do not drip the oil directly into the ear. Continue this treatment twice each day until symptoms disappear. If no improvement is noted within 72 hours, discontinue its use.

Halitosis

Halitosis, or "bad breath", is one of the most annoying and embarrassing of all human ailments. It is an extremely common condition, afflicting millions of Americans.

Clinical studies have documented tremendous value for tea tree oil in curbing halitosis. This makes sense, since bad breath is thought to arise as a consequence of microbial overgrowth in the mouth and tea tree oil kills microbes. When the microbes are killed the odor disappears.

To treat this condition apply the oil to the gum surfaces and also on the tongue. This should be repeated morning and night for one week. In most instances no other treatment will be necessary.

People who are constipated often have bad breath. This is particularly true of people who go several days without having bowel movements. In these instances the use of tea tree oil alone is insufficient, as it is important to diagnose and treat the underlying causes of the constipation. Normal bowel function must be established before the halitosis can be completely cured.

An alternative way to treat halitosis is to use antimicrobial mouthwashes. The public is familiar with advertisements for certain mouthwashes which claim to kill the germs that cause bad breath. Unfortunately, most of these mouthwashes use alcohol as their antiseptic, which is found in concentrations as high as 30%. Recent studies suggest that this alcohol content is toxic to the mucous membranes, particularly those of the oral mucosa, and that regular use of alcohol-based mouthwashes significantly increases cancer risks. In contrast, tea tree oil mouthwashes kill microbes without damaging the delicate mucosal tissues. Carcinogenicity is not a concern with topical use of the oil. Tea tree oil-based mouthwashes are the safest and most effective antimicrobial products for regular usage on the sensitive oral mucosa available on the market today.

Inflammatory Joint Disease

Diseases of the joints are among the most painful and debilitating of conditions afflicting Americans. Inflammatory Joint Disease is a categorization which includes osteoarthritis, rheumatoid arthritis, psoriatic arthritis, infective arthritis, bursitis and gout. Osteoarthritis, which afflicts millions of Americans, is the most commonly occurring of these. It is manifested by chronic inflammation of the joints and affects usually several joints primarily in the hands, shoulders, hips, spine and knees. In contrast, bursitis and gout usually affect only one joint and the inflammation tends to be more acute.

There are two common links between all of these conditions: joint pain and a reduction in mobility. In certain instances the joint is visibly swollen. However, in most cases pain and lack of motion are the dominating symptoms.

Tea tree oil is a topical anti-inflammatory agent with properties similar to salicylate-based liniments. It offers the advantage of exhibiting anti-inflammatory effects while acting as a topical anesthetic. Thus, it is of tremendous value in the treatment of virtually all types of inflammatory joint diseases, although it is particularly useful for the treatment of acute conditions. Often, there will be a visible reduction in the joint swelling within minutes after application. Additionally, it can be rubbed into sore and inflamed muscles, ligaments or tendons. For this latter usage tea tree massage oil is most beneficial.

Periodontal Disease

Also known as gum disease, periodontal disease is the plague of modern times. Over 90% of Americans have it, and some reports indicate that every one of us suffers with it to some degree. The extent of involvement varies from mild inflammation to severe gum recession and caries. Gingivitis, or inflammation of the gums, is the most common type of periodontal disease.

The gums are the bedrock which support and house our teeth. Gum disease is the predecessor of tooth decay. People with severe gingivitis are more likely to develop caries than those with relatively healthy gums.

There is little question that gingivitis is due largely to infection within the gum tissues. The problem in treating this condition relates to the difficulty in identifying specific causative organisms. Thousands of species of organisms reside within the mouth. Some are normal residents, while others are pathogens. Under certain circumstances the normal flora within the mouth may themselves become pathogens.

The gums are one of the toughest tissues within the body. Normally, they fit tightly against the teeth. They act as a barrier to infection. Once the gums become diseased, infection can more readily develop. Hundreds of pathogens are capable of infecting diseased gums. Ultimately, the pathogens destroy the tooth enamel, and, as a result, caries develop. Only certain pathogens are capable of eroding enamel, which is the hardest substance in the body. Yet, if the infection is prolonged, the enamel can be eroded all the way to the root of the tooth. The root (i.e. the nerve) is then easily infected. This may result in caries or what is commonly known as "toothaches."

Due to the plethora of organisms found within the mouth, only broad-spectrum antimicrobial agents are effective in the treatment of dental diseases. Tea tree oil meets this specification. Regular application reduces the total bacterial and fungal counts in the mouth. Studies have shown that it is highly active against numerous oral pathogens, including Candida, actinomyces, aspergillus, fusobacterium, peptococcus, bacteroides, pseudomonas, spirochetes and streptococcus.

Tea tree oil helps soothe inflamed gum tissues, and its regular application reduces the formation of plaque. It speeds healing of these tissues by destroying pathogens, and this allows local immunity to be restored. It is an ideal treatment for gingivitis with its symptoms of sore, bleeding and boggy gums. It helps reduce the pain and bleeding on contact. Regular application of the oil not only prevents gum disease but also helps restore normal function and structure to diseased gum tissue.

Dental Decay

The most serious dental condition is infection of the teeth and the roots of the teeth. Caries are responsible for the greatest degree of dental morbidity.

The dental anatomy makes infections of the teeth and roots difficult to eradicate. With root infections in particular, the problem in curing the infection is the difficulty in delivering the medicine to the infection site.

For decades dentists in Australia have utilized tea tree oil and continue to use it in the treatment of tooth decay. They add the oil directly to the cavity sites before and after drilling for fillings. They saturate tooth sockets with the oil after extractions. Australian dentists instruct their patients to apply the oil to diseased teeth several days prior to drilling or extracting in order to reduce post-surgical complications. Infection is the most common complication of invasive dentistry. An untold amount of suffering could be prevented if dentists applied tea tree oil before and after performing invasive procedures. Unfortunately, few American dentists are aware of tea tree oil's tremendous utility in this respect.

A study performed on tea tree oil was recently published in the dental journal *Periodontology*. The objective of the study was to confirm or dispel reports of the antimicrobial effects of tea tree oil on organisms known to cause dental decay. The researchers were astounded at their findings. Their conclusion: tea tree oil possesses significant antimicrobial action against oral pathogens. The researchers agreed that the pure undiluted and unrefined oil possessed the greatest antimicrobial activity.

To treat diseased teeth apply 2 to 3 drops of the oil directly to the enamel with a cotton swab three times daily after brushing. For gum disease apply the oil sparingly over the inner and outer gum surfaces morning and night. A small amount in toothpaste would act as an effective aid in the reduction of oral pathogens. A more convienient method is to rinse the mouth with tea tree oil mouthwash in the morning and at night.

Psoriasis

This skin condition afflicts up to 3% of Americans. Psoriasis is characteristically manifested by raised patches of inflamed, scaly skin usually red and/or white in color. These lesions are located primarily on the skin folds and exposed surfaces such as the knees and elbows.

Many drugs have been used to treat this condition, including sulfasalazine, cyclosporine, methotrexate, ketoconizole, vitamin D analogues and fish oils, all of which have demonstrated some degree of effectiveness. Corticosteroids are used topically to suppress the inflammation and growth of the lesions. One of the most common medical treatments is coal tar plus ultraviolet radiation, the use of which is declining somewhat due to concerns of toxicity. Most of these drugs exhibit toxicity, especially if used over prolonged periods.

Tea tree oil is not a cure for psoriasis. This condition is a systemic disease and topical treatments only scratch the surface. The central causes must be diagnosed and effectively treated before progressive improvement can occur.

Nizoral is one of the most effective treatments, and it is particularly useful for psoriasis of the scalp. However, it only temporarily represses the lesions, since, in most instances they invariably return as soon as the medicine is stopped.

The application of tea tree oil helps reduce the irritation

and inflammation of psoriatic lesions. When used in combination with prescription antifungal agents, it speeds the rate of lesion regression. It helps decreases scaling and itching while soothing pain.

Rashes

Tea tree oil is indicated for any itching rash. In most instances it will stop itching on contact. It is particularly useful in rashes due to contact with toxic plants such as poison ivy, sumac and oak. Rub on the rash a 5 to 10% mixture of tea tree oil in olive oil or use a 5% prepared cream several times daily. Tea tree oil helps neutralize the poisonous resins left on the skin and acts as a solvent to help remove these resins. This illustrates how valuable tea tree oil soaps are for washing skin contaminated by poisonous substances.

Rashes are usually caused by allergic reactions. These reactions may be localized, affecting one region of skin. Alternatively, they may be a manifestation of systemic disease. Infections may also result in them: for instance, the rashes of Lyme disease, Rocky Mountain Spotted Fever and Scarlet Fever. Rashes are one of the most common side effects of drugs and are descriptively known as "drug eruptions." They may also arise from sensitivity to soaps, perfumes, lotions, clothing fibers and/or jewelry.

Respiratory Diseases

It was mentioned previously that the Australian tea tree belongs to the same plant family as the eucalyptus tree. Plants of this genus are commonly found in New Zealand and Australia. The oils from these plants soothe irritated mucous membranes and help open blocked sinus and nasal passages.

For decades, oil of eucalyptus has been utilized in Western

medicine for the treatment of minor ailments of the respiratory tract. The use of tea tree oil for this purpose has only been more recent. However, it offers advantages that far exceed that of eucalyptus. In addition to opening closed respiratory passages, it helps kill the microbes that infect the throat, tonsils, sinuses and lungs. Stubborn respiratory tract pathogens, such as strep, staph, diphtheria, tuberculosis, pneumoccous, Candida, and pseudomonas, have been found to succumb it its antibiotic powers.

Tea tree oil is useful as an adjunctive treatment for a variety of bronchial and lung ailments, including bronchitis, pneumonia, influenza, whooping cough and croup. Additionally, it may be utilized in the treatment of acute and chronic sinusitis.

To treat these conditions inhale the oil several times daily. Alternatively, add it to a misting device or vaporizer. It may also be rubbed on the chest in a diluted form and can be mixed with petroleum jelly or, preferably, coconut oil. This will provide a steady release of the vapors overnight. These measures should be followed regularly until the infection clears.

Tea tree oil chest rubs are extremely useful for treating children with croup, flu or pneumonia. Always remember that these are adjunctive therapies to be applied in addition to treatment prescribed by physicians.

For sore throats and/or tonsillitis add 5 to 10 drops to a glass of water and gargle with this solution several times daily. Avoid swallowing, although small amounts accidentally swallowed in this dilution are harmless.

Seborrhea, Psoriasis, Eczema and Dandruff of the Scalp

Diseases of the scalp are common in America. Such diseases include seborrhea, psoriasis, eczema and simple dandruff. As diverse as these diseases might seem, they all have a similar origin, that being infective. It is a general rule that any condition involving flaking of the scalp and/or inflammatory scalp lesions possesses an infective origin.

Some of the most astounding evidence for this was brought forth by Rosenberg and cohorts of the University of Tennessee. These researchers established that even simple dandruff is associated with infection and that the scalp, hair follicles and sebaceous glands all may be infected. The primary culprits appear to be yeasts, but not Candida. Apparently a yeast that is a normal inhabitant of the scalp overpopulates under certain circumstances and causes flaking of the scalp. If the infection is prolonged and severe, eczema or psoriasis of the scalp may result. However, fungal infection is not the only causative factor. Nutritional deficiency plays a significant role, as does the type of diet. Additionally, Dr. Rosenberg found that certain bacteria may infect the scalp, notably staph and strep, and that these infections are common in patients with eczematous and psoriatic scalp lesions.

Nizoral cream has has been successfully for psoriasis of the scalp, and this is largely a result of its potent antifungal activity. While Nizoral is effective in the majority of cases, it is not a long term cure and its use carries the risk of systemic toxicity even if applied topically. Hepatotoxicity (liver damage), as manifested by elevation of liver enzymes, occurs in as many as 10% of users. Thus, liver enzymes must be monitored whenever patients are placed on this drug.

Tea tree oil contains numerous terpenes which are highly fungicidal, but these are poorly absorbed. In contrast to Nizoral cream, topical application of small doses of tea tree oil will not cause hepatotoxicity. The molecules of tea tree oil stay primarily on the skin, where they are needed most.

For the treatment of scalp disorders apply the diluted oil directly to the scalp or saturate the scalp with a 5 to 10% solution of tea tree oil and olive oil. Leave overnight and cover with a nightcap. Repeat daily for up to one month.

Tea tree oil may be used in shampoo for dandruff control.

Add two teaspoons of oil per eight ounces of shampoo. After lathering, wait at least one minute before rinsing.

Dandruff is an exceedingly common condition, and nearly one half of Americans have it. It is an annoying as well as embarrassing ailment.

Tea tree oil shampoos out-perform most over the counter dandruff shampoos in achieving long-term cures for this condition. For best results shampoo the hair daily for one week. Rinse thoroughly with a dilute solution of water, tea tree oil and vinegar. As a maintenance use the shampoo two or three times weekly. Daily use of any shampoo over prolonged periods may weaken the immunity of the scalp and increase the risks for scalp infection.

Seborrheic dermatitis is yet another scalp illness caused by chronic infection of the scalp. In most instances both bacterial and fungal infections are involved. This condition is manifested by heavy scaling and flaking of the skin. Involved regions include the face, scalp, hands, feet and torso. Thus, it can occur on virtually any region of the body.

Nutritional deficiency is a contributing cause of seborrhea. Deficiencies of vitamin A, biotin, vitamin B-2 (riboflavin), vitamin B-6 (pyridoxine), essential fatty acids, zinc, sulfur and selenium have all been documented, and treatment with these nutrients invariably results in improvement.

In particular, the development of seborrheic dermatitis is a sign of severe essential fatty acid deficiency. Zinc, B-2, B-6 and biotin are all required for optimal digestion and utilization of essential fatty acids.

Itching and flaking of the skin (or scalp) are common symptoms of seborrhea. Excessive itching may lead to excoriation with resultant secondary bacterial infection. When this occurs the infection may enter the hair follicles in which case it would contribute to hair loss. In fact, hair loss is a common symptom of severe seborrhea of the scalp. In order to restore optimal hair growth, the infection must be destroyed. To achieve this create a 10% solution of tea tree oil in

Balancing Infusion, and apply it to the scalp every evening before bedtime. Do this regularly until the infection and scaling clears. Then apply the solution three times per week for preventive purposes. Balancing Infusion is a blend of essential plant oils, and it contains the essential fatty acids so desperately needed by the skin cells of the scalp (to order call (800) 243-5242).

There is an additional benefit of this treatment: improved hair quality. Fungal infection of the scalp chokes the flow of nutrients to the hair follicles. The result is that the hair shaft is weaker and, often, the infection actually causes and/or perpetuates hair loss. The cosmetics of the hair and scalp will usually improve if the infection is eliminated. Thus, the results of the tea tree oil/Balancing Infusion treatment may include the following:

1. improved hair texture
2. stronger hair shafts
3. increased thickness
4. reduction of hair loss
5. elimination of dandruff and seborrhea
6. relief of itchy scalp

Tea tree oil by itself is not a cure for seborrheic dermatitis. Yet, its application usually relieves the annoying symptoms of flaking, as it represses the growth of causative microbes. It can be applied directly to the lesions or used in shampoos. When applied directly on inflamed lesions a temporary burning sensation should be expected.

Optimal results are achieved when antimicrobial treatment is combined with nutritional therapy. The diet should be high in natural fats and protein and low in sugar, particularly refined sugar. Daily doses of essential fatty acids, zinc, selenium, vitamin A, B-6, biotin and riboflavin should be taken.

Pruritic (itchy skin)

Itchy skin is certainly annoying, yet it can also be an indication of serious disease. However, usually it is a manifestation of relatively minor ailments such as allergic reactions or dry skin. Diseases/illness which may cause pruritis include:

hepatitis
cancer
kidney infections
kidney failure
liver failure
food allergies
contact allergies due to poisonous plants, soaps and metals
internal fungal infections
skin fungal infections
essential fatty acid deficiency
vitamin A deficiency

Tea tree oil is one of Nature's finest anti-itch remedies. Often, it relieves the itching on contact. Apply tea tree oil creams and lotions to the involved site(s) several times daily. Alternatively, mix a 50/50 solution of tea tree oil and olive oil and rub into the skin. In most instances the itching will be relieved immediately. However, if no improvement is noted within a day or two, consult your physician.

Sports Injuries

The number and variety of injuries that can occur in sports is immense, especially combat sports such as football and hockey. Injuries to the joints and ligaments are the most common type seen. An additional type of injury is trauma to the soft tissues.

Soft tissue injuries are defined as trauma to the skin, fatty tissue, cartilage and muscle. Included are cuts, bruises, abrasions, contusions, strains, sprains and muscle pulls/tears.

The primary utility of tea tree oil in sports is as an antiseptic and anti-inflammatory agent for use on open wounds and sores. Here it will prevent microbial contamination of the injury site. It may also prove useful when applied on injuries resulting from blunt trauma such as bruises and contusions.

Tea tree oil may be applied in the field to contaminated wounds. This will help prevent minor wounds from developing into serious ones due to infection. It is ideal for use on large abrasions which are contaminated with dirt. Often, these wounds are impossible to clean adequately in the field, as the dirt is compacted into the wound. Saturating the wound with tea tree oil will assuredly prevent infection and will greatly enhance the rate of healing.

It is rare that a game of basketball, baseball, football or hockey is played without at least one player suffering a cut, abrasion or other open wound. In basketball, games are played on a floor coated with human sweat and other secretions. Abrasions and cuts are common. It is easy to comprehend how open wounds could become contaminated by microbes, sweat, saliva and even by blood from other players. In football, games are often played on artificial turf. Usually, numerous players suffer abrasions from impact on this harsh synthetic grass. These abrasions are extremely painful. Washing them with water makes them sting, let alone antiseptics, which may produce unbearable pain. In contrast, washing the wounds with tea tree oil, even the undiluted oil, is usually sting-free. In fact, it cools the painful wounds while sterilizing them and helps cleanse them of debris. No other antiseptic can offer the benefit of killing infection while actually decreasing pain.

The "Magic" Johnson revelation has shaken up the entire world, although the impact will probably be greatest in the world of sports. A healthy, powerful athlete, a role model for millions of children, teenagers and adults has become infected with the AIDS virus. While intimate sexual contact remains the primary mode by which this virus is spread, the contraction of

HIV infection by Mr. Johnson serves as a stark reminder of how vulnerable humans are regardless of their health or social status. For athletes this news is scary. The question is now arising: Could the AIDS virus be transmitted from one athlete to another via combative contact? Could a non-infected athlete develop HIV from a wound that becomes contaminated with blood or saliva from an infected person? There are no such cases on record. However, there are several cases where health care professionals have infected patients with HIV---or visa versa---although this contact is no less significant than that between athletes in sports. In fact, the propensity for contamination may in some instances be even greater in these sports than that between doctors and patients. The fact that no cases have yet been reported is no cause for laxness: Who would have ever thought that Magic Johnson would have developed HIV?

Tea tree oil kills numerous viruses as well as other microbes which contaminate open wounds. Its capacity for preventing viral contamination of wounds is greatest if it is applied immediately after the injury.

The odds for transmission of infection are directly related to a concept called "contact time." This is defined as the period of time where the noxious organisms are in contact with the open wound before cleansing or antisepsis is applied. Open wounds bleed; that is not the problem. The problem is that whatever contaminates the wound may be shuttled back into the body. The shuttle system can be descriptively called the *reverse circulation*. This is a natural process whereby the body relieves the wound of toxins, contaminants and, yes, microbes. There are two systems of reverse circulation: the venous blood vessels and the lymphatic vessels. Both are capable of rapidly absorbing and distributing microbes from the contaminated region into the general bloodstream. From here the microbes may gain entry to virtually any organ or tissue in the body.

If a wound is left untreated, the microbes which contaminate it will likely replicate and infect the region by the billions. Innumerable microbes may gain entrance into the bloodstream. In normal individuals the immune system will fight the infection. It will attempt to wall it off and prevent the microbes from entering the bloodstream. However, viruses, in particular, have numerous ways of eluding the immune defenses. HIV has the ominous attribute of invading the very white blood cells which are produced to destroy viruses. It parasitizes them, taking over their cellular machinery. HIV causes the ultimate type of cellular toxicity: it overpowers the cell's genetic mechanism and literally controls its every move. Then it kills them.

Tea tree oil can sterilize fecal matter, which is essentially nothing but microbes. Nearly 90% of the solid weight of the stool consists of microorganisms. An acutely contaminated wound is certainly much less of a challenge for tea tree oil's antiseptic powers compared to raw feces. Repeated application of tea tree oil to the wound will result in complete or near complete sterilization. This knowledge may save lives, since evidence is accumulating that HIV and other life-threatening pathogens may be transmitted through direct inoculation into open wounds.

Hopefully, aggressive antisepsis will become a mainstay for all injuries occurring during contact sports events. At a minimum wound infection will be prevented, and that alone will be beneficial for the players and the team, as pain will be curbed and the rate of healing greatly enhanced. In any case, why take chances?

Tea tree oil has other uses in sports. It is a topical anesthetic and anti-inflammatory agent. Thus, it can be applied on all types of strains or sprains. Here, it may act to decrease swelling and numb pain. This diversity of uses makes it clear that a bottle should be kept in every athletic trainer's bag.

The Dog Bite Oil

As incredible as it may seem, over a million people are bitten by dogs every year. The Postal Service is well aware of the scope of this dilemma, as thousands of mail carriers are included among the victims. The extent of this problem is so vast that bites by other animals, including cats, must be considered relatively rare in comparison. In fact, human bites are the second most common "animal" bite.

Any animal bite can readily become infected. This is because bites are a type of puncture wound where contaminated secretions are injected deep into the tissues. Deep wounds receive less oxygen and other important healing nutrients from the blood than do superficial ones. Blood flow is greatest in the skin and least in the deep muscles. This reduced blood flow largely contributes to the high risk for infection in puncture wounds.

Dog bites are notorious for becoming infected, and the rule of thumb is that any dog bite which breaks the skin, no matter how superficial, will become infected. In emergency rooms physicians advise patients to leave dog bites open and rarely suture them. Experience has proven that closing (suturing) the wound will serve to hold the infection within the tissues . Not only will the wound heal poorly if it is closed but also potentially severe or even life-threatening infection may result.

Tea tree oil is a godsend to the dog bite victim. It penetrates deep into the punctured, scuffed and/or bruised tissues, killing pathogens immediately. Repeated application will prevent infection from developing in most instances. To treat dog bites, first wash the wound thoroughly with water and an antiseptic soap (tea tree oil soap would be ideal). Next, saturate the wound with tea tree oil. Repeat this treatment at least three times daily for several days. Then apply tea tree oil once per day until healed.

Any type of breakage in the skin could potentially become infected. Such open lesions respond positively to tea tree oil's antiseptic powers. Thus, it is ideal for application on acute injuries such as superficial cuts, wounds and/or abrasions. Tea tree oil is also invaluable for infusion into puncture wounds of all types in order to prevent serious infections from developing.

CHAPTER 3

Fungal Diseases

The incidence of fungal diseases in America has risen dramatically in the past 20 years. The scope of this problem is so great that according to some authorities, infections by fungi are reaching near epidemic proportions.

There are thousands of species of fungi. Only a small percentage of these infect humans. One of the most common human pathogens is Candida albicans. This yeast can infect virtually any tissue or organ in the body. Other pathogenic fungi include the dermatophytes, which infect the skin and nails, and lung pathogens such as aspergillus, histoplasma, coccidioides, pneumocystis and blastomyces.

One of the greatest concerns with fungal infections is the fact that all pathogenic fungi are capable of suppressing immune function. Previously, it was thought that fungi only infect patients whose immune function is already suppressed and that such infections are rare in healthy individuals. Now it is known that fungi can infect anyone from newborns to healthy adults.

Many theories have been advanced to explain the mechanisms behind the immunosuppressive effects of fungi. Some authorities believe that this is due to the liberation of fungal toxins which poison the immune system. They point out that the fungi are capable of secreting specific chemicals which impede the function of immune cells. Some of these chemicals have been found to prevent white blood cells from replicating. The chemicals also prevent white blood cells from phagocytizing fungi. Other researchers believe that fungal cell wall components are the primary culprits which impair immunity. Whatever the mechanism might be, the existence of chronic fungal infection is synonymous with debilitated immune function.

Fungal infections represent an added burden upon the immune system, which is already overwhelmed by a host of other stresses. These stresses include chronic and acute infections, exposure to toxic chemicals, drug therapy, impaired nutrition and emotional stress.

Pathogenic fungi are highly invasive and are capable of infecting virtually any tissue within the body, including the skin, lungs, liver, spleen, thymus, adrenal glands, intestines, rectum, pancreas, stomach, bladder, kidneys and even the brain. The most common sites of infection are the skin, mucous membranes, nails, bladder, intestines and lungs. The extremities, particularly the hands and feet, are the most likely sites of skin fungal infections. The mucous membranes are, in a sense, extensions of the skin and are readily infected by a variety of fungi, although Candida albicans is the most common culprit.

It seems astonishing that the stomach, which secretes the most caustic and potent acid known, can become infected by fungi. The upper portion of the stomach and the lower esophagus in particular are frequent sites of Candida infections. The development of these infections is encouraged by the consumption of acid-suppressing drugs. Such drugs include Tagamet, Zantac and antacids. Long term usage of these drugs causes a profound depression in the synthesis of stomach acid, which is one of the most important natural defenses against infections. The prolific usage of these drugs is a major reason that esophageal candidiasis is so common today.

Stomach acid kills microbes. Without it, the esophageal and/or stomach mucosa are readily infected by Candida and a host of other pathogens. In fact, under these conditions Candida can infect the entire gastrointestinal tract from the mouth to the anus. Other substances or factors which lead to a suppression in the production of stomach acid include folic acid and B-12 deficiency, meatless diets, alcohol consumption, cigarette smoking, smokeless tobacco, antibiotics, cortisone, non-steroidal anti-inflammatory agents and aspirin.

Additionally, refined carbohydrates encourage the growth of fungi and yeasts. So do birth control pills, especially if they are taken chronically. The estrogens found in these pills enhance the growth of yeasts.

Recent research indicates that the amount of dietary carbohydrate consumed, particularly refined sugars, influences the pathogenicity and adherence of yeasts. Those who consume massive amounts---the per capita consumption in the United States is nearly 130 pounds per person per year---are at the greatest risk. The growth of other fungi, such as those which infect the skin, are also encouraged. All yeasts and fungi are sugar loving, as sugars are their primary food.

The food supply in America is laced with refined sugars. These sugars are added to a wide range of foods. There are no nutritional benefits from this sugar-lacing. In fact, the added sugar detracts from quality nutrition. Refined sugar consumption induces deficiencies of a wide range of nutrients, including biotin, riboflavin, thiamine, niacin, pyridoxine, pantothenic acid, folic acid, vitamin C, chromium, manganese, magnesium, calcium, potassium, copper and zinc.

Individuals who suffer from chronic fungal infections should carefully read labels to determine if refined sugars are added to the foods. Refined sugars which are commonly added to processed foods include corn syrup, maple syrup, invert sugar (levulose), molasses, cane sugar (also called white sugar and/or sucrose), beet sugar, dextrose, maltose, honey (cooked or refined), fructose and glucose.

In addition, certain fruit juices consist almost entirely of sugar. These include orange, apple, grape, cherry and pineapple juices. Yeasts feed ravenously off of these natural sugars, which may stimulate their growth just as readily as refined ones.

The labeling of certain foods as "sugar-free" is misleading. This is because, while they may not contain cane sugar, they are sweetened with sugars derived from other sources such as raisin extract, apple juice, pear juice, grape sugar, fructose and/or honey.

A primary characteristic of yeast infection is the existence of tissue invasion. That is why chronic infection by Candida is descriptively called *mucocutaneous candidiasis*. In other words, Candida albicans causes chronic, difficult to treat infections by invading superficial tissues such as the skin, nails, nail beds and mucous membranes. Candida is able to accomplish this through the secretion of tissue destroying enzymes and the production of mycelia, tiny thread-like extensions which invade tissues, cells and cell membranes.

One of the major obstacles in eradicating Candida infections, as well as other fungal infections, is getting the medicine to penetrate deep enough into the site of the infection. If a person weeds a garden by mowing the weeds only, they will grow right back. The cure is achieved by digging the weeds out by the roots, or, in today's age, destroying the roots with chemicals. In a similar manner it is crucial to utilize medicines which penetrate as deeply as possible into the skin and mucous membranes. This is precisely the advantage of tea tree oil. It has the greatest penetrating capacity of any known antifungal agent. As it saturates the tissues, it kills fungal organisms on contact.

Tea tree oil exhibits excellent penetration in epithelial tissues. These tissues include the skin, gums, nails and mucous membranes. It is the treatment of choice for stubborn fungal infections of these regions. It is able to deliver its medicinal chemicals directly through the innumerable cracks and crevices found throughout the mucous membranes and skin to the site of infection. By doing so tea tree oil effectively attacks deep seated, resistant fungal infections.

Chronic yeast infections are reaching epidemic proportions largely as a consequence of the prolific use of broad spectrum antibiotics. Antibiotics are prescribed by physicians all over the world, and billions of pounds of them in the form of syrups, pills or capsules are consumed yearly. Evidence exists that the consumption of antibiotics in food---our fish, red meat, poultry, eggs and milk products are tainted with them---encourages the overgrowth of Candida albicans and other fungal pathogens.

Candida albicans: A Cause of Chronic Disease?

Candida albicans is a commensal organism, which means that it is found normally in humans and plays a specific role as one of thousands of indigenous gut flora. These various species of microbes exist in a delicate balance, one which is easily disrupted by antibiotic therapy. The fact is antibiotics decimate the normal flora, most of which are bacteria. The significance of this is a result of the fact that their natural role is to inhibit the growth of pathogenic organisms. When the inhibitory bacteria are destroyed and Candida populates the tissues in large numbers, that is when physiological damage occurs.

Researchers have discovered that Candida albicans damages tissues through the secretion of enzymes as well as a variety of chemical toxins. Many of these chemicals are waste products or by-products of the yeasts' metabolism. These by-products include the highly toxic chemical *acetaldehyde*. This compound causes inflammation and, in the extreme, tissue destruction.

A wide range of conditions have been associated with yeast overgrowth. These conditions include:

acne
AIDS
arthritis
cancer
chronic bronchitis
chronic fatigue syndrome
Crohn's disease
constipation

cystitis
diabetes
eczema
esophagitis
food allergies
intestinal malabsorption
irritable bowel syndrome
lupus
migraine headaches
pneumonia
prostatitis
psoriasis
sinusitis
ulcerative colitis
urethritis
vaginitis

The elimination of Candida infection leads to great relief in symptoms and an improvement in overall health. Nothing is more irritating for women than a severe case of Candida vaginitis or for men Candida prostatitis.

Men and women pass this organism back and forth between themselves through sexual contact. Women develop symptoms most easily, and the infection is more common in men than is medically recognized. In men, infection may be manifested by symptoms of prostatitis: urinary urgency, incomplete voiding, frequency and urethral discomfort.

Yeast infections are particularly common in uncircumcised males. Itching of the penile head, discharge, foul odor, redness and urethral discomfort are the usual symptoms. If symptoms of genital or urinary tract infection exist and no bacteria are cultured, infection by Candida should be suspected even if the yeast cannot be cultured.

Tea tree oil is not a treatment for internal fungal infections. However, for fungal infections of the skin and mucous membranes, it is the treatment of choice. It is ideal for use in the ultra-sensitive genital regions and, in most instances, will not cause irritation or side effects.

Vaginitis

Every day millions of women suffer with vaginitis and vaginal discharge. Much of this disability is caused by Candida albicans. Other fungi may play a role, and bacteria also represent a major cause. However, Candida is the most common culprit in terms of a single organism.

The incidence of vaginitis has greatly accelerated over the last 30 years. This is largely the result of the extensive usage of prescription antibiotics. Candida albicans should be presumed the cause of vaginitis in women who develop vaginitis and/or vaginal discharge while or shortly after taking a course of antibiotics.

Antibiotics destroy the normal bacterial flora which inhabit the vaginal and intestinal mucous membranes, allowing fungal organisms to overpopulate. These fungi, which include numerous species of Candida, cause a deep-seated vaginal and/or intestinal infection which is difficult to eradicate.

Vaginitis is among the most common complaints of females visiting doctors' offices. It is more common than PMS. In some clinics nearly one-half of the office visits are accounted by women afflicted with it.

What is even more disturbing is that a majority of these women fail to be cured. Thus, the condition usually persists despite the use of the typical anti-bacterial and anti-mycotic medications.

Those suffering with severe inflammation of the genital regions may notice a temporary stinging or irritation after applying the pure oil. In such instances it is advisable to utilize the antiseptic cream, which contains 5% tea tree oil by volume, or tea tree oil suppositories.

Vaginitis is a generalized term. Therefore, it encompasses

a variety of vaginal problems, including inflammation, irritation and infection. The infections include those caused by parasites, bacteria, fungi and viruses or a combination of these. Irritation and inflammation may be caused by chemicals found in sanitary napkins, tissue paper, tampons, perfumes and bubble baths. The excessive use of soap within the vaginal tract commonly results in vaginitis, since the mucous membranes within the vagina maintain a delicate balance of pH and secretions, and harsh soaps upset this balance. Most soaps and bubble baths are basic in pH; the vaginal tract is slightly acidic. Thus, soaps alter the pH toward basic. This increase in pH weakens the delicate vaginal immunity, and infection is a common consequence.

The type of clothing worn may influence vaginal health. Of greatest importance is the type of underwear. Those containing synthetic fibers, such as nylon and polyester, are most detrimental. Synthetic fibers emit noxious chemicals, such as formaldehyde, which compromise the function of vaginal immune cells. When the vaginal immunity is impaired, the overgrowth of noxious organisms is encouraged. Additionally, synthetic underwear fail to allow "breathing" and, as a consequence, cause the retention of moisture within the vaginal region. This trapped moisture encourages the growth of yeasts. What's more, synthetic underwear tends to retain organisms even after washing. As a result individuals can become re-infected by their own clean underwear. Underwear made from natural fibers are the safest to wear. While these underwear do contain residues of chemicals as a result of dying and bleaching, the chemicals are readily washed out. What's more, microbes and the organic matter they thrive on are more easily cleansed from natural clothing. Additional disinfection can be accomplished by adding half a teaspoonful of tea tree oil to the wash cycle. Ideally, wash the underwear in a separate load.

What is most important about natural fibers is that they allow for breathing. This means that the skin of the pubic region and the mucous membranes of the vagina will obtain adequate oxygen from the environment and release waste gases as well as moisture. Remember, synthetic underwear holds moisture tightly against the body. If this moisture retention occurs on a daily basis, fungal and/or yeast infection is virtually assured.

Poor hygiene and the degree of sexual activity also play significant roles. So does age. Additionally, vaginitis may be caused by the excessive use of douches. Many women douche regularly on the basis that they are doing something good for their bodies. However, routine douching dilutes protective vaginal secretions, and this may actually increase the risks for infections. Routine soaping and douching of the inner vaginal membranes is one of the most common practices predisposing individuals to the development of vaginal irritation and/or vaginitis.

Symptoms of vaginitis include odor, irritation, itching, spotting, pain and discharge. These symptoms are often exacerbated during menses. Pregnancy may precipitate vaginitis, particularly yeast vaginitis, since the increased amounts of circulating estrogens encourage the growth of yeasts. It is important to eradicate the pregnancy-induced vaginitis, particularly if it occurs late in pregnancy, in order to prevent transmission of the infection to the infant during delivery.

For decades physicians have sought to remedy vaginitis through the application of topical medicines applied within the vagina. These medicines include antibiotics, antimycotics, salves and anti-inflammatory agents. Cortisone, the most potent anti-inflammatory agent known, is a component of many vaginitis medications.

Bacterial, viral, parasitic and yeast infections all can cause vaginitis. So can allergic reactions, chemical toxicity, spermicides, drug reactions, excessive douching and excessive soaping. However, it is usually difficult to determine the exact cause of vaginitis. In terms of overall incidence, bacterial infections appear to dominate, and there are literally hundreds of species which can infect the vagina. Consequently, medical researchers have searched for that broad spectrum drug which acts as a cure all, a substance which "kills everything." That is why Flagyl is currently being used as a topical treatment for vaginitis. This philosophy is understandable. Researchers discovered many years ago that the causative organisms of vaginitis are difficult to culture, and this makes the establishment of a definitive diagnosis tenuous. Plus, in the usual case, several organisms are involved. Even when there is a high level of suspicion that the primary cause is yeast infection, the organism is not always cultured and infections by other organisms may complicate the problem.

Physicians, as well as researchers, have encountered great difficulty in their attempts to make a specific diagnosis for this condition. This is so much the case that they have stated that in the case of bacterial vaginitis, definitive recognition of the organism is "not helpful." The greatest obstacle to achieving a definitive diagnosis of bacterial vaginitis is the fact that these organisms exist in such vast numbers---by the billions---in the vaginal tract. Plus, hundreds of different species normally inhabit it.

Often, a variety of bacteria simultaneously infect the vaginal mucosa. That is why the current treatment for bacterial vaginitis is so precarious. No species specific antimicrobial agents can be given. Thus, broad spectrum antimicrobial drugs are usually prescribed. However, this therapy is inadequate, since potent medicines cause numerous side effects, which may be of a worse nature than the infection itself. In a sense the use of antibiotics for the treatment of bacterial vaginitis amounts to a sort of "Hail Mary" hit or miss approach in the treatment of this complicated disease.

Antibiotics exacerbate vaginal candidiasis. In fact, a large percentage of cases of vaginal candidiasis occur directly as a result of antibiotic therapy. Thus, susceptible women might develop candidiasis of the vagina while or shortly after taking a course of prescription antibiotics.

The usual symptoms are a white cottage cheese-like discharge combined with intense itching. Candida vaginitis can exist without these symptoms. However, it is rare that it will occur without the existence of at least some sensations of itching or irritation. If itching, irritation and a white discharge exist, the diagnosis is virtually confirmed.

Chronic or recurrent candidiasis often develops in diabetics, birth control pill users and individuals taking antibiotics over prolonged periods. Pregnant women are often afflicted with it, and those with multiple pregnancies are most vulnerable. It may even be present in otherwise healthy individuals. Additionally, women who regularly use cortisone or prednisone, whether topically or internally, are at a high risk for the development of mucosal candidiasis.

Trichomonas Vaginitis

Vaginal trichomonas infection is caused by the flagellated protozoan *Trichomonas vaginalis*. This organism has a propensity for infecting the sexual organs, notably the vagina, uterus, prostate, seminal vesicles and urethra.

Trichomonas is one of the most commonly occurring sexually transmitted diseases, and it afflicts millions of Americans every year. Symptoms are highly variable, although with vaginal infection there is usually one characteristic sign: a frothy discharge. In males the infection is often difficult to diagnose, and no symptoms peculiar to this organism are found. They are usually treated only as a consequence of the diagnosis in female sexual partners.

Treatment consists of Flagyl. Sexual partners must be treated simultaneously, and abstinence from sex during the course of treatment is advised. Flagyl is not the safest drug to use, but it is the most effective one. The consumption of alcohol must be avoided during treatment, and Flagyl should be avoided during pregnancy. Care must be taken to explain side effects, particularly with women of child-bearing years.

Tea Tree Oil: Broad Spectrum and Effective Cure for Vaginitis

Tea tree oil is of immense value for the treatment of vaginitis. It is just as effective as the standard antimicrobial agents utilized to treat this condition. What's more, it has none of the systemic side effects of Flagyl or other broad spectrum antibiotics.

Regular use of diluted or properly prepared tea tree oil usually results in a cure regardless of the types of organism(s) involved. However, its greatest utility is seen with yeast vaginitis, although it is highly active against trichomonas as well. Its anti-yeast powers are largely due to its ability to penetrate deep into the vaginal mucosa. This mucosa consists of numerous layers, and Candida is capable of invading all of them. This deep invasion is why Candida vaginitis is often difficult to cure through the use of standard anti-fungal agents, which are incapable of completely penetrating the vaginal mucosa. This is also why the infection recurs so frequently after treatment. In contrast, the deep penetrating action of tea tree oil results in a more complete kill of the yeasts than can be achieved with other medicinal substances.

Much of tea tree oil's value as an antiseptic agent is a consequence of its ability to destroy a wide range of organisms, and this attribute makes it ideal for the treatment of vaginitis. Remember, vaginitis is a garbage can diagnosis, and the organisms which cause it are so numerous that an all-inclusive list has yet to be developed. Another advantage of tea tree oil is that vaginal pathogens are unable to develop resistance to it.

Treatment of vaginitis with prescription antibiotics may be necessary, especially if evidence for the existence of specific bacterial or fungal infections exists. However, there is always the risk of inducing Candida vaginitis if the prescriptions contain antibacterial agents and/or cortisone. In this instance, the patient is sent from the frying pan to the fire.

Many vaginal creams contain cortisone. Even in small quantities cortisone depresses vaginal immunity. Additionally, it thins the vaginal mucosa making the establishment of infection more likely, since the normally thick vaginal mucosa acts as a barrier against infection.

It is true that cortisone often helps relieve itching and other distressful symptoms of vaginitis. Yet, at what price? While the symptoms are suppressed, the vulnerability to both acute and chronic infections is increased. Cortisone is known particularly for enhancing the growth of yeasts and fungi. In contrast, diluted tea tree oil reduces inflammation, decreases or eliminates itching and curbs pain safely without impairing immunity or damaging the delicate vaginal lining.

Every day millions of women throughout the world suffer with this debilitating condition. However, much of this suffering is needless.

Tea tree oil is the only antiseptic which is capable of eliminating each of the major types of vaginal infections, while exhibiting virtually no toxicity to vaginal tissues. To treat vaginitis saturate a tampon with a 10 to 20% solution of tea tree oil mixed with extra virgin olive oil. Replace the tampon after 4 hours. Or, simply apply the olive oil/tea tree oil solution to the vaginal walls three or four times daily. Tea tree oil suppositories are also available. These offer the advantage of being easy to administer; plus, they are portable.

The Invasive Nature of Fungal Infection

According to Dr. Mahmoud Khanam of the University of Kuwait, a noted microbiologist, the key to the success of pathogenic organisms in infecting human tissues is the ability to implant. This represents the organism's capacity for invading the tissues deeply enough that it establishes its existence permanently. In this manner microbes can infect the skin, mucous membranes and even the internal organs. Once microbes invade the tissues they begin to multiply and may soon overwhelm the capacity of the immune system to destroy them. That is when significant chronic infections begin.

Without such penetrative ability microbes would simply be washed through our bodies or would fall off our skin. That is what makes fungal infections so difficult to eradicate. Fungi are capable of penetrating deep into the tissues through highly specialized methods of tissue invasion. They secrete potent proteolytic enzymes, which destroy and/or damage cellular membranes. In addition, the fungi produce hyphae which are, in essence, fungal tentacles. These tentacles invade human cells off of which they feed, deriving various nutrients such as sugars, vitamins and minerals. Thus, they harm the cells both by direct damage to the cell membranes and also by depriving them of the nutrients they need to survive.

Candida albicans is probably the most well known and heavily researched example of an invasive pathogenic fungus. A single organism is capable of producing dozens of tentacles. Once Candida latches onto the tissues it is difficult to eradicate. Its tenacity has confounded medical researchers and physicians alike, who have attempted to destroy it with everything from potent antifungal agents to nuclear radiation.

Evidence points to immune stimulation as the most effective and efficient cure for internal fungal infections. Candida infection cannot develop in individuals with strong immune systems. Thus, even if exposure occurs, a healthy immune system will prevent infection from developing.

In studying Candida researchers have gone to the extreme of infecting healthy volunteers the organism. The yeasts proceeded to invade the bloodstream and internal organs. Then they were cultured from these regions. However, within a matter of hours yeasts could no longer be cultured, indicating that the immune systems of these individuals efficiently cleared the organisms from the tissues. Unfortunately, in today's era a great many people are afflicted with compromised immune function. What's more, even the healthiest of immune systems may find the battle overwhelming, especially if massive inoculation occurs.

Clearing Chronic Fungal Infections: What are the Benefits?

The term chronic means long term. Thus, chronic infections are those which have existed for weeks, months or even years. Such infections persist despite attempts by the immune system to eradicate them.

Human beings are parasitized by a variety of pathogens, which disrupt optimal health. All of these parasites cause immune stress when they infect humans chronically.

Yeasts and fungi commonly cause chronic infections in humans. As many as 30% of Americans are afflicted with chronic fungal infections of some sort. While our immune systems may adjust to their existence, these infections diminish our well being and usually cause annoying symptoms.

A great deal can be accomplished as a result of the successful treatment of yeast and/or fungal infections, even localized ones such as athlete's foot. Curing these infections takes a tremendous load off the immune system. In a sense the riddance of the chronic infections means there is one less thing for the immune system to deal with and a burden is lifted from the mind as well, since these infections are often disfiguring and disheartening.

People who suffer with chronic fungal infections often exhibit symptoms of other complaints, as most are plagued with ill health. Included are digestive ailments, low blood sugar, chronic fatigue, vulnerability to colds and flu, chronic headaches and even mental disturbances. These conditions are frequently aggravated by chronic fungal infections and, in certain instances, may even be caused by them.

Women who have yeast vaginitis endure intense and often

prolonged suffering. Many have been treated medically for weeks or months to no avail. This is the ideal opportunity to utilize a natural treatment, especially one that works quickly and consistently.

Infection by Candida albicans is particularly known for its chronicity and tenacity. Thus, it is one of the most difficult of all infections to eradicate. Like other pathogenic fungi, Candida albicans invades the mucous membranes through a phenomenon called *germ tubule formation*. Germ tubules are microscopic finger-like projections which bore into the skin or mucous membranes in search for food. The primary food required by yeasts is sugar. Germ tubule formation plays such a critical role that without it, significant infection is impossible. Once adherence occurs the infection moves into the phase of being chronic. At this point it is nearly impossible to eradicate it.

Most medicines fail to destroy those yeasts which have invaded deep into the tissues. Tea tree oil is the exception. The oil can penetrate deeply into the infection site, completely saturating the involved tissues with its curative components. Regular application blocks the formation of germ tubules, while destroying existing yeasts.

Tea tree oil is an effective treatment for all types of vaginitis, including that due to trichomonas, which is notoriously difficult to treat. In 1962 a study was published in Obstetrics and Gynecology showing astonishing results in Trichomonas vaginitis. The treatment consisted of saturating tampons with tea tree oil and using them as suppositories. Additionally, tea tree oil douches were applied. In 1985 Dr. Belaiche of the University of Paris performed a study on 28 patients with chronic vaginal candidiasis. Before and after scrapings documented a significant improvement in all cases. Nearly 75% of Belaiche's patients achieved a complete cure despite experiencing poor results previously with standard antimycotic agents.

One of the greatest attributes of tea tree oil as an antifungal agent is that fungi are unable to develop resistance to it. Unfortunately, the same cannot be said regarding prescription and over the counter antifungal agents. Resistance to Nystatin is common, and it may develop with ketoconizole and myconizole as well. In contrast, tea tree oil can be applied repeatedly for months or even years, and no resistance will develop. With many standard antifungal agents as soon as the medicine is withdrawn, the infection comes raging back. At this point the organisms may have developed into resistant strains. In other words, although their growth is suppressed by the drugs, no kill is achieved.

Drug-resistant strains of yeasts are usually difficult to eradicate, and, while repeated applications of prescription medicines may suppress their growth, achieving a complete cure may be impossible. This is not so with tea tree oil. Its complex molecular nature and peculiar mechanism of action makes it virtually impossible for microbes to develop resistance to it. Thus, one of its greatest values is in the treatment of antibiotic-resistant vaginitis. It can be used alone or in combination with standard therapy to achieve an aggressive destruction of the organisms.

Is Chronic Candidiasis Real?

Many doctors are skeptical about the existence of the syndrome of chronic candidiasis. Some go so far as to claim that it doesn't exist. Others admit that it exists but insist that it only occurs rarely and in individuals whose immunity is severely depressed. Yet, as many patients know, the condition is very real.

Numerous researchers have documented the existence of mucocutaneous candidiasis as a condition afflicting millions of Americans. These researchers have found that chronic candidiasis can develop both in immune compromised and otherwise healthy individuals. What's more, they have determined that there is a clear cut relationship between antibiotic usage and the onset of mucosal candida infection. The fact is antibiotic therapy is the primary cause of this condition, as these drugs greatly enhance the invasive powers of yeasts.

One of the most profound problems in establishing the existence of chronic candidiasis is the fact that only overt infections can be diagnosed by standard methods of culture and sensitivity. Thus, in the majority of patients the annoying symptoms persist even though doctors are unable to establish a firm diagnosis.

Even when the infection is severe, Candida may be difficult to culture. Doctors usually assume that negative cultures preclude the diagnosis of yeasts as the primary cause of illness.

Currently, physicians recognize that symptoms and medical history are the most crucial components for establishing the diagnosis and determining the appropriate treatment. Tests are performed only for confirmation. Wouldn't these same principles hold true for yeast and fungal infections?

Long-term use of antibiotics causes a suppression of cellular immunity. This is the type of immunity involving the function of white blood cells. These cells are the front line defense against infections. Additionally, antibiotics destroy the normal bacterial flora which are found in large numbers within the bowel, vagina and on the skin. These flora are responsible for inhibiting the growth of pathogens on the skin and mucous membranes. They are particularly active in preventing yeast overgrowth. Additionally, the normal flora produce a variety of antibiotic-like substances which specifically inhibit the growth of yeasts.

Evidence for the existence of the syndrome of chronic candidiasis is extensive; it is not a psychological disease. Millions of Americans are afflicted with it. Chronic yeast infections are responsible for significant morbidity, and women, in particular, are affected. Additionally, those taking antibiotics, birth control pills or cortisone are at added risk for its development. Symptoms of chronic candidiasis include:

* intestinal bloating
* indigestion
* heartburn
* diarrhea
* constipation
* coated tongue
* intestinal gas
* allergies
* cravings for sugar
* fatigue
* sinus problems
* anxiety
* mood swings
* depression
* PMS
* menstrual cramps
* vaginitis
* insomnia
* cold extremities
* headaches
* pruritus

Oral Candidiasis

Also known as oral thrush, this condition is seen relatively rarely. However, its incidence is rising significantly in the United States. The key to understanding its rarity is in the usage of the term "seen." In other words, to see the white patches in the mouth which are distinctive of this condition is rare, that is to see them in adults. However, subclinical infection of the oral mucosa by Candida is relatively common in adults. The gums, tongue and throat may become infected without the presence of discernable white patches.

The existence of oral thrush is significant, as it may be a sign of serious underlying disease. However, it also develops in otherwise healthy individuals, including newborns, infants and pregnant women.

One of the major factors involved in the rising incidence of oral thrush is the AIDS epidemic. Many AIDS victims initially present with oral candidiasis. A majority of these individuals also have rectal and/or vaginal candidiasis. Another major factor in the causation of oral thrush is the increasing usage of immunosuppressive drugs, including chemotherapeutic agents, broad-spectrum antibiotics and cortisone.

Tea tree oil is an effective cure for oral thrush. In appropriate strengths, it may be prescribed for newborns, infants, teenagers and adults. However, only a 5% dilution is recommended for repeated use in pregnant women, as some transmission of the oil through the skin may occur.

Tea tree oil can be used in conjunction with systemic anti-fungal therapy. Such therapy must be prescribed when treating immune-compromised individuals, such as AIDS and cancer patients, who present with oral thrush as their initial symptom. That is because oral thrush represents only the tip of the iceberg, and it is likely that systemic infection by Candida exists. In severe cases the internal organs are infected, including the liver, spleen, intestines, esophagus, stomach, adrenal glands, bone marrow, bladder and kidneys.

Direct application of the diluted oil to the involved tissues, such as the tongue and oral mucosa, usually relieves pain and eliminates itching. While oral thrush is one of the most difficult infections to cure, repeated application of tea tree oil eventually results in eradication of the lesions. Individuals with sensitive mucous membranes may need to apply a dilute solution of 10% or less. Tea tree exhibits potent antifungal activity even in these dilutions.

Fungal Infections of the Nails

The nails are living tissues which are highly active metabolically. They are essentially an organ system in themselves with their own unique nutritional and biochemical needs.

Despite their obvious hardness, the nails are vulnerable to becoming infected by a host of organisms, although the primary culprits are the fungi. Several fungi can infect the nails as well as the nail beds and folds (the nail folds are defined as the soft tissues surrounding and encasing the nails).

The two major categories of nail infections are those of the soft tissues, or nail folds, and those of the hard surfaces, which includes the nails and nail beds. Nail fold infection is known medically as *paronychia*; that of the nail and nail bed is called *onychomycosis*. Technically, onychomycosis is defined as fungal infection of the nail, while, with the term paronychia, no specific type of causative organism is implied.

Most toenail and fingernail infections are caused by fungi. In contrast, the majority of infections of the nail folds are due to bacterial invasion. Paronychia is more specifically defined as inflammation and infection of the soft tissues surrounding the nails; the most common causative organism is staphylococcus. However, some researchers maintain that Candida is the primary cause, although the greatest weight of evidence places it as a secondary invader.

Primary bacterial infection of the nails is rare. However, fungi readily infect them. The dermatophytes are the most aggressive pathogens which attack the toenails. Other fungi which cause nail infections include Candida, aspergillus and scopularlopsis brevicaulis. Nails damaged by fungi are readily infected by bacteria, and pseudomonas is one of the most common culprits. These *secondary infections* are usually easily eradicated; it is the primary fungal infections which present the greatest challenge.

The dermatophytes, notably trichophyton

rubrum/interdigitale and epidermophyton, cause the majority of toenail infections. These infections usually begin in the aftermath of severe cases of athlete's foot. The fungi initially infect the skin of the feet, often gaining access through wounds or cuts. In most cases the infection begins between the fourth and fifth toes, where moisture is often retained. The existence of moisture on the skin greatly enhances the invasiveness of these fungi, which have difficulty parasitizing dry skin. Most dermatophyte infections develop in individuals who utilize locker-room type facilities, where the organism thrives in moisture-laden areas.

Once the fungi gain entrance through the skin the infection is spread throughout the entire foot, particularly the sole and between the digits. Next, the fungi invade the nail bed. The first sign of infection is a thickening along the lateral margin of the nail. Often, only one or two toes become infected. In other instances all of the toes are involved. Usually, toenail infections begin at the lateral margins and then spread to affect the entire toenail.

The treatment of toenail fungus constitutes tea tree oil's most astounding use. No other substance, whether synthetic or natural, can match it. Toenail fungal infections are notoriously difficult to cure and are, in fact, regarded by medical authorities as incurable. This thinking may be more due to ignorance than pessimism. Apparently, the medical profession is unaware of the powers of Australian gold; tea tree oil has been proven effective for this condition. In fact, if the oil is regularly applied to the involved nail(s), the achievement of a partial or complete cure is almost certain. It may take several weeks or months before a complete cure is attained. Rapid improvement is often observed in infected fingernails and also the nails of the small toes. However, larger nails, such as those of the thumb and great toe, may take an exceedingly long time to improve. In this regard it is important to remember that these are chronic infections which have likely been in existence for months or even years prior to initiating treatment.

Tea tree oil is capable of penetrating the deepest layers of the nail and nail bed. It is important for the antifungal medicine to achieve this penetration, since the nail bed, which is located under the nail and skin, is the seat of the infection.

Fingernail infections are occurring with increasing frequency, particularly in women. This is largely a consequence of the use of various chemicals on the nails such as fingernail polish and polish remover. Glues, such as those used on artificial nails, also contribute to the increased incidence. They contain solvents which destroy the structural integrity of the nail bed. Additionally, the artificial nails themselves increase the risks for yeast infections of the nails. That is because these nails prevent normal air exchange within the nail bed. When this occurs moisture is trapped, which encourages fungal overgrowth.

Candida is regarded as the most frequent culprit with fungal infections of the fingernails. Candidiasis of the nails is usually manifested by white patches or a lifting (thickening) of one edge of the nail plate. Subsequently, the mycotic infection may spread to involve the entire nail and nail plate.

To treat this condition saturate the nail and nail bed with tea tree oil twice daily. In case of severe fingernail infections, four applications daily may be necessary.

Athlete's Foot

Athlete's foot is a fungal disease which afflicts millions of Americans and not just athletes. It is caused by *dermatophytes*, fungi which have a propensity for infecting keratin, the protein which makes up our skin, hair and nails. These fungi cause a variety of infections classified as *tinea*. Tinea capitis refers to fungal infection of the scalp; tinea barbae, of the beard; tinea corporis, of the trunk and extremities; tinea cruris, of the groin; and tinea pedis, of the feet. Ringworm is another term used to describe these infections.

The causative organisms invade human skin through the secretion of potent enzymes capable of eroding the skin. They may also invade and infect the hair follicles as well as the sebaceous glands.

Once skin fungal infection becomes established, it is extremely difficult to eradicate. The immune system nearly always fails to eradicate it on its own. This is because chronic tinea causes an impairment of local as well as systemic immunity. If the infection is severe enough, secondary infection by a variety of bacteria will occur. These bacteria include pseudomonas, staph and strep, all of which further suppress the immune system. Additionally, Candida albicans commonly infects skin or nails damaged by tinea.

Athlete's foot and the associated toenail fungal infections are bothersome chronic conditions which are difficult to cure. Standard medical treatments include antifungal creams/sprays and oral antifungal agents such as griseofulvin.

Tea tree oil contains a number of compounds which are highly active against the fungi which cause athlete's foot. It is more effective for the treatment of foot and toenail fungal infections than griseofulvin. If the two are used simultaneously, the dosage of griseofulvin may be lessened. This is important, since griseofulvin may be toxic to the liver. Liver enzyme function must be monitored during therapy with this drug.

Tinactin and similar over the counter antifungal remedies are effective treatments for athlete's foot but are impotent in curing toenail fungal infections. Plus, they are much more costly than tea tree oil. Tea tree oil's greatest advantage is a consequence of its unique ability to penetrate human skin, which allows it to reach the primary sites of infection: the dermal layers and the nail bed.

Even the most stubborn cases of athlete's foot infection usually respond to tea tree oil therapy. This is best exemplified by a case history. One man was recently cured of athlete's foot fungus infection of nearly 50 years duration. He contracted the infection during World War II while stationed in the tropics. As he had a relatively severe case, he tried virtually every known antifungal remedy to no avail. Finally, he discovered tea tree oil. Regular application of the oil cleared the infection completely within days.

For optimal results apply the oil liberally on the involved region twice daily. In the case of stubborn infections three to four applications daily may be necessary. Additionally, the oil may be added to a warm foot bath: use one teaspoon per quart of water and soak for one-half hour.

Jock Itch

No single organism can be held responsible for this distressing condition. However, the most common culprits are various yeasts and fungi. That is why tea tree oil can bring such dramatic relief for this condition.

The skin folds are common sites of fungal infections. This is largely because moisture is retained within the folds, since contact of skin against skin holds moisture in. Skin is living tissue which breathes. This breathing, which amounts to the exchange of gases and moisture with the air, keeps the skin dry.

Fungi are moisture loving, that is they thrive in moist environments. Although fungal pathogens of the skin, such as trichophyton and epidermophyton, are the most common culprits which cause jock itch, yeasts, including Candida, may also be responsible. Additionally, bacteria may secondarily infect the groin, particularly if it excoriated.

Tea tree oil possesses antimicrobial activity against all of these organisms. It is a reliable cure for jock itch. The application of tea tree oil usually results in immediate relief of the itching. It surpasses all other remedial agents for this condition in terms of rapidity of results, symptom relief, cure rate and cost effectiveness.

To treat jock itch apply tea tree oil twice daily to the involved region. For optimal results apply only on dry skin. Additionally, the 5% cream preparation is ideal for the treatment of this condition.

CHAPTER 4

Nature's Insecticide

With the exception of microorganisms, insects are the most pervasive and numerous of the creatures on this earth. As a result insect bites commonly occur, and not just in the wild. They happen frequently right in the home and backyard.

Insects continue to inhabit every crevice and corner of this earth despite man's unrelenting attempts to destroy them. Whether an individual lives in the tropics, desert, plains, mountains or North Pole, he/she will encounter them. Certainly, there are regions where a person is at a greater risk of being bitten: for instance, the forests of the Northeastern and Northwestern United States and the subtropical regions of Florida. Here, in moist environs and under the cover of lush forests, insects abound in great numbers. Yet, even in the most barren stretches of land they can be found in significant numbers, actively creating whatever mischief they may. All kidding aside, insects are far from evil. As difficult to believe as it might be, all species of insects serve useful functions, even cockroaches.

Bites by insects are often innocuous. However, they may also result in serious allergic reactions and/or infections. Although rare, death can result.

Bites and stings are more likely to become infected if the organism secretes venom or saliva into the tissues. An additional means by which bites/stings result in infections is if parts of insects are left in the skin. The existence of these remnant parts, known medically as foreign bodies, nearly always leads to localized infection. People who have had splinters that couldn't be removed know how true this is. Invariably, the region surrounding the splinter becomes infected. The same is true when insect parts, such as stingers and pincers, are embedded within the skin.

Tea tree oil is invaluable as a treatment for insect bites. Those accustomed to its utility, such as the Aborigines and Australian bushmen, regard it as a cure-all. This attribute is most deserving, since it can be used as a treatment and/or antidote for virtually any type of bite, wound or sting resulting from insects or any other biting creatures.

The application of tea tree oil to the bite helps sterilize the remnant parts of the insect and prevents the development of localized infections. It neutralizes venom from bites by wasps, bees, fleas, mosquitos, centipedes and spiders. More potent venoms, such as those from snakes and scorpions, may also be neutralized. Additionally, it reduces the inflammation and swelling that results from these bites.

Immediate application of tea tree oil is crucial when dealing with bites by dangerous insects or animals. This will help reduce the risks for venom-induced allergic reactions. These reactions are the most common cause of death from insect bites. The oil should be applied repeatedly if a significant bite occurs. Its penetrating action allows it to saturate the wound site and, thus, neutralize the venom before it can enter the systemic circulation. Serious bites still require anti-venom treatment in case the venom has travelled throughout the body.

Most biting insects carry pathogenic microbes in their saliva. These microbes include viruses, bacteria and parasites. For instance, malaria is caused by parasites, and mosquitos are the carriers. The mosquitos inject malarial parasites through their saliva when they bite. In the case of Yellow Fever viruses are the pathogens, and they too are injected into skin through the bites of mosquitos. Bacteria are the culprits with Lyme disease and are carried in the saliva and excrement of deer ticks. Encephalitis may be caused by a virus carried by mosquitos, the virus originating from the blood of horses. Typhus fever is caused by a bacteria-like organism called *Rickettsia* which is transmitted to humans through the bite and excrement of lice or fleas.   Mite larvae transmit the bacteria which cause *Scrub Typhus*, a condition seen primarily in Southwest Asia, Australia and the Pacific islands.   Thus, it is not the bite itself with which to be most concerned; it is what is transmitted by the bite.   It is the risk for the development of infection after the bite that is most ominous.   That is why tea tree oil is so valuable.   Its timely application will prevent the onset of systemic infection by killing the microbes on contact.

People who frequent the outdoors should be well supplied with this versatile oil.   Fishermen and swimmers would be pleased to know that leeches don't stand a chance if tea tree oil is applied to them: they simply fall right off the skin.   This capacity was well known to Australian bushmen, who were frequently attacked by leeches as they traversed the swamps. Tea tree oil is the bushman's medicine cabinet in a bottle, but it is also the golfer's, swimmer's, fisherman's, hunter's, hiker's, mountain climber's, bird watcher's, camper's,......

Ticks, Ticks, Ticks: Paranoia or Plague?

While researchers have documented that tea tree oil neutralizes a variety of insect venoms, just how it does so is unknown. Why the oil is toxic to insects is also a mystery.   Insects with pincers will immediately retract and fall off when tea tree oil is applied to them, leaving behind no pincers, fangs or stingers.   This makes tea tree oil an ideal remedy for bites caused by one of America's most feared insects: ticks.

Ticks belong to the same insect family as spiders: the arthropods.   They are notorious for infecting humans and other mammals by clamping tightly into the skin with their powerful pincers.   They can attach anywhere in the body, but the most likely site is on the scalp.   A significant number of diseases are transmitted via the bites of ticks. These diseases include Lyme disease, Rocky Mountain Spotted Fever, Tick Typhus and Q-fever.

Tea tree oil is exceptionally effective against ticks. Application of the oil causes the tick to retract its pincers and fall harmlessly off the body. Alternatively, the oil may kill it on contact.

If a tick is found attached to human skin, it and surrounding tissues must be saturated with the oil until the tick dies or retracts. Even if the tick falls off it is important to saturate the skin surrounding the bite with tea tree oil repeatedly in order to prevent the spread of infection. In case the tick bursts, wash the area thoroughly to remove tick parts, saliva and excrement. Then saturate the involved region with the oil. This treatment will neutralize any toxins secreted by the tick and will kill the tick-borne microbes responsible for Lyme disease and other serious infections.

The odds for being bitten by ticks is far greater with individuals who venture into the wilderness than for city dwellers. No sportsman, naturalist or adventure seeker should be without tea tree oil when in the wild. Additionally, the oil should be stored in the glove compartment of the auto and also at home.

Lyme Disease: Illness on the Rise

The incidence of Lyme disease has risen exponentially over the last decade. In part, this may be due to heightened awareness of the existence of this relatively new disease and also improved methods of diagnosis.

Lyme disease is caused by a bacteria called *Borrelia burgdorferi*. This bacteria infects humans through the bite of ticks, notably deer ticks. This tick, which is exceedingly small, is so named because deer act as its primary carriers, although other mammals may carry it as well.

Even with the current heightened awareness, the signs and symptoms of Lyme disease may be difficult to recognize. This is because it mimics many other conditions. Indeed, it is one of the most bizarre and unpredictable diseases known. Only a peculiar rash fully distinguishes it from other conditions, and this develops in less than 50% of patients. More commonly, symptoms such as fatigue, malaise, headaches and joint pain are seen. The problem is that these symptoms are found in numerous illnesses. What's more, most patients cannot recall being bitten by ticks or, for that matter, any other type of insect.

In most instances this infection is mistakenly diagnosed as a bad case of the flu or a cold. Only later does it become known that the symptoms are due to Lyme disease, and that is usually well after the infection becomes firmly established.

In a sense, the wrongful diagnosis of Lyme disease as cold or flu syndromes represents an error in clinical acumen. Certainly, the characteristic rash which occurs with Lyme disease is not a common symptom of colds or flu. A thorough history should lead the physician to suspect a condition other than the common cold. Lyme disease usually occurs during the summer months when ticks are most active. Rarely does it happen in the late fall or winter when the incidence of colds and flu is the greatest. This rule applies to the Midwest and Eastern states. In temperate regions, such as California, Lyme disease may develop year around. Additionally, the infections occur most commonly in the Northeastern states as well as Georgia, Michigan, Wisconsin and Missouri. The states with the highest incidence are New York, New Jersey and Wisconsin. It rarely occurs in Montana, Nebraska, Arizona, Colorado and Florida. Despite these clues, the diagnosis of this bizarre and elusive disease may be missed even by the most astute clinicians.

Today there is a sort of paranoia, if not hysteria, concerning Lyme disease. The chronically ill read about this illness and often attribute their symptoms to this condition. In most instances Lyme disease is not responsible for their illnesses. Despite this fact, many of these individuals consult numerous physicians in hope that evidence can be procured for a positive diagnosis.

While it is true that the tiny ticks which cause Lyme disease are difficult to spot, tea tree oil can be applied to any suspect lesions that might develop after wilderness adventures. Plus, tea tree oil shampoos can be used to wash pets, particularly dogs, which may act as carriers for the ticks. A person doesn't have to be in the wild to contract this disease: golfers get it as do executives and housewives. Pets which frequent the outdoors can bring the tick right to the home.

Rocky Mountain Spotted Fever

Rocky Mountain Spotted Fever (RMSF) is a serious and potentially fatal disease. Like Lyme disease, RMSF is carried by ticks, although they are larger ones than those which transmit Lyme disease. It is also carried by mites. The ticks and mites transmit a highly infectious bacteria-like organism called *Rickettsia*.

This illness received its name from the fact that it was first reported in the Rocky Mountain states, notably Montana and Idaho. Currently, it occurs with greatest frequency along the Eastern coast and in the Appalachian states. Here, there is a virtual epidemic of this tick-borne illness in certain segments of the population. In the last 20 years the incidence of this illness has more than tripled. Mortality rate is high compared to other infections; in some regions it may reach 10%.

Rocky Mountain Spotted Fever has been reported in every state in the USA as well as in Canada and South America. Currently, the greatest number of cases are reported in Maryland, Virginia, Georgia, North Carolina, Tennessee and Oklahoma. In the Eastern states dogs act as the primary carriers of the ticks. Thus, people living in the aforementioned states who develop the symptoms of Rocky Mountain Fever and who are in close contact with canines must be suspected of having the disease. If a high level of suspicion exists, doctors should immediately perform the appropriate lab work, which includes complete blood chemistry, blood cell counts and antibody levels for Rickettsia. Additionally, canine contacts should be checked for the presence of ticks. A thorough physical exam should be performed on patients, which includes searching for evidence of the tick or its infection site. In most instances, no tick can be found. If an attached tick is discovered it must be removed with the utmost care, never forcibly. The easiest and safest way to remove it is to apply generous amounts of tea tree oil. Invariably the tick will either fall off intact, die and be easily removed, or rupture. If the latter happens, the site of rupture must be immediately cleansed after which tea tree oil should again be applied. Continue to apply the oil to the wound or bite site several times daily for at least three days to insure destruction of any remaining organisms.

Symptoms of RMSF include sudden onset of headache, fever, chills and abdominal pain. These symptoms usually last from 2 to 3 weeks.

Every year, thousands of individuals are bitten by the ticks which cause RMSF. However, only a relatively small percentage of these individuals develop the illness. Transmission of the disease is unlikely unless the tick remains attached for several hours or days or is removed forcibly. An additional mechanism for infection is the forcible removable of the ticks from dogs. If ticks are crushed, fluids and/or feces from the ticks may contaminate the individuals hands. Unless the hands are washed immediately afterward, transmission of the disease is likely. RMSF is diagnosed most easily once the initial period of infection has elapsed. This is because the most characteristic signal of the infection is the development of a peculiar rash which usually arises on or about the fourth day. Initially, the rash is found on the extremities: the wrists, ankles, palms, soles of the feet and forearms. Within 24 hours, it extends to the rest of the body, including the face. If these symptoms develop a physician should be consulted immediately.

Antibiotics are the treatment of choice for Rocky Mountain Spotted Fever. Tetracyclines are most often used, since they exert specific action against rickettsial organisms. Other antibiotics are ineffective; in fact, they may exacerbate the condition.

Despite the advent of antibiotic therapy, RMSF leaves its mark in terms of causing prolonged illness and/or mortality. This may be due to the fact that in the case of Rickettsia, antibiotics at best inhibit the organism's growth. In other words, tetracycline cannot kill the organisms outright. However, a healthy immune system can effectively destroy them, and everything possible must be done to support and stimulate immune function. Nutrients which enhance immune function include vitamin A, vitamin C, vitamin E, pyridoxine, pantothenic acid, folic acid, zinc, copper, selenium and manganese. Many Americans are deficient in these nutrients. Recent studies have shown that as many as 80% of Americans recieve in their diets less than the RDA for such nutrients as folic acid, zinc, copper, manganese and vitamin A.

An additional problem is the fact that Rickettsia are increasingly developing resistance to tetracyclines. This emphasizes the value of the timely application of tea tree oil to the tick and/or bite region to help prevent further dissemination of the microbes.

If a tick is found latched to the body, call your physician immediately. Then apply tea tree oil. Do not attempt to remove the tick forcibly. Application of the oil will neutralize the tick's poisons and prevent further infection. If the tick fails to fall off, have it removed by medical personnel. They may wish to save the tick to have it analyzed.

Pharmacies and health food stores, particularly those in the states with a high incidence of RMSF, should keep a stock of tea tree oil readily available. It should be purchased by outdoorsmen and kept in their backpacks and vehicles.

Pets commonly carry ticks as well as a variety of other insects. The hands should be thoroughly washed after handling pets. When shampooing them be sure to use a tea tree oil shampoo or add several drops of tea tree oil to the shampoo. Regular use of these shampoos will help prevent dogs and other pets from acting as carriers for ticks.

Head Lice

Nothing creates more anxiety in parents or school teachers than an outbreak of head lice. It is an embarrassing illness to contract, and, traditionally, a difficult one to eradicate. Hardly a year goes by without some local school experiencing an outbreak of it. According to the Center for Disease Control (CDC) approximately 10% of all elementary school children are treated for lice infestations each year. In these outbreaks dozens and often hundreds of children may become infected. In some instances the entire student body may suffer the infestation.

Lice infection is easily spread. Children act as vectors, spreading it directly to other children by close contact and indirectly through contact with contaminated objects.

Head lice infection, known medically as *pediculosis*, is spread by the translocation of the eggs of the louse from one human to another. The organisms live by attaching themselves to hair shafts, where they deposit their eggs. Then they burrow into the scalp. Additionally, lice may attach to the axilla, torso or pubic region, that is any region covered with hair.

Invasion of the scalp leads to inflammation and intense itching. When children itch the region(s) they get the eggs of the lice on their hands and under fingernails. Then they contaminate the rest of their bodies, other children and various objects with the eggs.   This is the primary way that the infection is spread.

If lice infect the scalp the itching can become so severe that people scratch right through their skin.   Researchers believe that it is the deposition of the lice excrement within the scalp which causes the inflammation and resultant intense itching.   Once the skin is excoriated, secondary infection by bacteria can easily develop.

Children are infamous for failing to adhere to appropriate hygiene.   One of their most common hygienic deficiencies is failure to wash their hands after utilizing the rest room.   They get dirt and other filth on their hands and often touch other body parts, itch their hair and even eat without washing the contaminants off.   This is a major reason that infections are spread so readily among children existing in close quarters.

Treatment

Over the last thirty years the primary medical treatment for lice infestation has been the use of potent insecticides similar to those used to kill pests.   Currently, malathion is added to anti-lice body shampoos.   Usually, one application of these shampoos is sufficient to achieve complete eradication.

All insecticides are potentially toxic, even in small amounts.   Researchers have found that trace amounts of insecticides impair the function of the immune, nervous and digestive systems.   It is not only internal consumption with which to be concerned; insecticides are just as readily absorbed when applied to the skin.   In fact, research published in the *American Journal of Public Health* indicates that skin absorption of pesticides and herbicides is several times greater than intestinal absorption.   Thus, regarding the treatment of head lice, a non-toxic topical treatment must be offered to the public so that parents have the option to choose between the natural and the toxic.

One of the major concerns with the use of insecticides for the treatment of head lice is that children have a smaller surface area compared to adults. This means they are more likely to absorb a relatively greater amount of the insecticide into their tissues than adults. Thus, children can more easily become intoxicated by these poisons. Plus, they are more vulnerable to the occurrence of severe, life-threatening allergic reactions. For these reasons, physicians should consider prescribing less toxic anti-lice drugs than those currently being dispensed.

With tea tree oil shampoos allergic reactions are far less likely to occur than with insecticides. The oil is infinitely safer than malathion; thus, shampoos containing it can be applied repeatedly without the concern of toxicity. With malathion, concerns for toxicity are so great that only a single application is recommended.

One mechanism by which tea tree oil clears lice infestations is through its solvent action. Its probable mechanism of action is that it dissolves the lice eggs on contact.

In the case of infection wash the entire body with shampoo fortified with two teaspoons or more of tea tree oil. Rinse the hair with a hot water solution containing an additional half teaspoon of the oil plus one tablespoon of apple cider vinegar. The hot water/vinegar helps dissolve the eggs and aids in the penetration of tea tree oil. After drying, saturate the comb with the oil and run it through the hair. Metal combs are preferable, as their stiff bristles help dislodge the eggs from the hair shafts.

Body and pubic lice infections are caused by the same organism which causes head lice. Pubic lice is more commonly known as "the crabs." Tea tree oil shampoos are equally effective for each of these conditions.

Remember, the superiority of tea tree oil over synthetic insecticides lies in its mechanism of action: it dissolves the lice eggs on contact, preventing further reproduction of the organism. It also kills existing organisms. Lastly, it has the unique attribute of achieving the desired results without harming human cells.

Public Concern Over Insecticides

Today, people are wary of insecticides and rightfully so. These chemicals have contaminated every part of the universe. Even the rain water contains measurable amounts.

Tea tree oil kills insects, and so it can technically be called an insecticide. However, it does so without damaging the environment. Additionally, it exhibits none of the toxicity characteristically seen with the use of chemical insecticides.

Insecticides have only one purpose: to kill pests. However, their fatal effects harm more than just insects. Every day thousands of animals and innumerable plants die as a consequence of insecticide toxicity. Evidence is accumulating that certain human diseases, such as cancer, multiple sclerosis, muscular dystrophy, Alzheimer's disease and Parkinson's disease, are caused by insecticide exposure. Thus, the use of potent insecticides for the treatment of illness should be avoided, whether in humans or animals. In fact, any usage of these compounds in the treatment of disease is dubious. This only makes sense. Agents which cause disease should not be used to treat it.

Scabies

Scabies is an infectious disease of the skin caused by the mite, *Sarcoptes scabiei*. It is highly contagious and may be contracted directly via exposure with infected individuals or indirectly through contact with bedding or other inanimate materials.

The Scabies mite infects humans by burrowing into the skin. Here, it lays eggs and reproduces. These burrows are most commonly found between the digits and on the palms, fingers, wrists and genital regions.

Scabies is manifested by intense itching and inflammation at the site of the lesions. The inflammation, which can be significant, is a consequence of the immune reaction against the entrenched organism and the toxins it secretes.

The standard treatment for scabies is similar to that for lice infestations: insecticides. Tea tree oil can be used instead and is equally effective. Its application leads to immediate relief of the itching and reduction in the inflammation. Tea tree oil is highly toxic to the scabies mite, and is particularly toxic to its eggs, which are destroyed even by dilute solutions. Regular application kills mites without the toxicity resulting from the use of chemical insecticides.

CHAPTER FIVE

The Personal Hygiene Antiseptic

Are the terms hygiene and cleanliness synonymous? Indeed they are. Hygiene is a method of cleanliness for the maintenance of excellence in health.

It was approximately 140 years ago that surgeons failed to wash their hands prior to performing their tasks and that doctors neglected to wash their hands prior to delivering babies. A lack of attention to hygiene was then responsible for the high rate of morbidity and mortality for maternity and surgical cases. Today, doctors thoroughly scrub their hands up to their elbows and don sterile clothing as well as gloves. Attention to hygiene is at its pinnacle in today's surgical suites.

However, in the general public there is a lack of adherence to careful personal hygiene. Carelessness in regard to hygiene is a major factor in the spread of infectious disease. Recent studies indicate that this is perhaps the number one factor leading to the spread of infectious diseases from one human being to another. The significance of this problem is illustrated by the numerous outbreaks each year of food poisoning in restaurant clientele. The most likely source is the failure of food preparers to properly wash their hands after using the rest room.

Most Americans believe that they cannot properly clean themselves without soap. While rinsing the body or hands with water alone will reduce bacterial counts, larger amounts of bacteria and filth will be removed if soap is used. However, this is true only of fresh bars of soap.

Recently, researchers discovered that used bar soaps may

actually contaminate the skin with additional bacteria. This is particularly true if several people use the same bar of soap. It seems that bacteria feed off the soap, which consists largely of organic matter. Thus, a single bar of soap may be contaminated by billions of microbes. For this reason pump soaps are far more hygienic than bar soaps and are the preferable type for use in hand washing, particularly in public places.

The ideal soaps would be those which contain antiseptics. The antiseptic content helps prevent the growth of noxious microbes within the soap and also reduces the bacterial count on the hands.

Tea tree oil soaps have been found to be as much as 60 times more powerful in killing various bacilli than other disinfectant soaps. Depending upon the amount of tea tree oil found in the soap, microbial counts may be reduced to nil.

One study done on hand washing showed the bacterial counts of unwashed hands were reduced more than 1000-fold by simply rinsing the hands with tea tree oil. This underscores the merits of the routine addition of tea tree oil to liquid pump soaps. Think of the value this would have in preventing the spread of infection. It would be exceptionally helpful for hand washing in children. They are constantly contaminating their hands and often fail to wash them after playing outdoors, eating and/or using the rest room. Tea tree oil soaps are the ideal agents for washing hands after performing potentially contaminating tasks such as changing diapers, cleaning toilets, handling pets or touching human secretions, i.e. blood, saliva, sputum or pus.

To enhance antisepsis add two teaspoons of tea tree oil per twelve ounces of pump soap. If the hands become contaminated with blood, fecal matter or infected secretions, additional antisepsis can be accomplished by rinsing the hands with the pure oil and water.

Prevention

Another valuable use for tea tree oil is the prevention of infection.   Certain individuals are susceptible to the development of recurrent infections.   This is certainly true of acne sufferers.   Some of these individuals suffer from unrelenting acne lesions on the face, upper back, neck and chest.   These lesions are not only annoying and embarrassing but may lead to disfiguring scars.   Men with heavy beards who shave frequently are susceptible to boils and acne-like lesions of the face or neck.   Women who shave their legs or underarm regions may develop boils and/or infective rashes.   Certain women are vulnerable to the development of boils and/or infected cysts in the vagina.

Other recurrent infections include staphylococcal boils, paronychia, jock itch and ringworm.   The routine use of tea tree oil soaps and/or massage oils may help prevent these infections from developing.   A tea tree oil lotion or cream can be rubbed on the potential infection sites.   Or, simply apply the undiluted oil, massaging it into the skin after bathing or showering.

The After Sex Lotion

In today's age doctors, lay people, school administrators, mayors, governors, senators and the president of the United States have one goal in common: preventing the spread of sexually transmitted diseases.   The medical and political professionals know full well that a significant problem exists. However, the Magic Johnson revelation has brought this to a precipice.

The fact that germs can be spread by close human contact is no secret. The question is can anything be done to prevent it?

The incidence of sexually transmissible diseases has

reached crisis, if not epidemic, proportions. The seriousness of the AIDS epidemic needs no repetition here. The incidence of syphilis is rising significantly, seemingly on parallel to that of AIDS. Gonorrhea is on the rise, and several highly pathogenic antibiotic-resistant organisms have been discovered. Chlamydia infection is exceedingly common and is a cause of significant morbidity in females and, to a lesser degree, in males. Infections by sexually transmissible viruses are perhaps the most feared of all venereal diseases. They too are rising in incidence. Included are HIV, HIV-like viruses, herpes and genital warts.

Infection cannot develop simply from exposure to the pathogen. The organism must become established within the tissues and must overwhelm local as well as systemic immunity. In short, it must develop a home front and maintain that existence against efforts by the immune system to destroy it. Thus, one key element for halting the transmission of sexually transmissible diseases is to prevent the organism from gaining entrance to the body, in other words, to prevent it from entering the bloodstream or internal organs. This emphasizes the value of the timely application of tea tree oil to the genital regions.

This is not to ignore the primary cause of venereal diseases: sexual promiscuity. The rising tide of sexually transmitted diseases can only be ebbed when this crucial issue is adequately addressed. Without proper programs to curb promiscuity, the use of tea tree oil amounts to little more than sprinkling water drops into a raging ocean.

Other Diseases

Hundreds of diseases may be related directly or indirectly to poor hygiene. Since the turn of the century, diseases due to poor sanitation/hygiene have diminished greatly. This was largely a consequence of the improvements in public sanitation.

Some physicians and researchers attribute the decrease in communicable diseases to the widespread use of immunizations. However, there is little support in the scientific literature for this claim.

The massive drop in incidence of communicable diseases, such as polio, influenza, cholera, dysentery, pneumonia, smallpox and diphtheria, is primarily a result of improvements in public sanitation: cleaner water and land; fewer rats and mice; running water and refrigeration. In comparison, immunizations played a lesser role. Certainly, the decline in the incidence of cholera, pneumonia and dysentery in this country cannot be attributed to immunizations. Nor have immunizations decreased the incidence of influenza. In fact, epidemics of this illness continue to rage the country despite our "sanitary" existence and flu vaccines.

All diseases of poor sanitation have one thing in common; they are transmitted from one human to another via close contact. They may be transmitted sexually. However, the most common mode is via human hands. In fact, the hands transmit more cases of communicable diseases than any other type of contact. Additionally, inanimate objects, such as toothbrushes, glasses, dishes, utensils, jewelry and even clothes, may be responsible for transferring pathogenic organisms from one human being to another.

The old adage is true; people can "catch cold" from other individuals, and this is especially true of those whose immune systems are impaired.

Germs may be picked up from objects, people, beverages and/or food. Is this cause for paranoia? Not at all. Tea tree oil kills germs generically. Thus, it comes to the rescue by killing the germs which may be found on people or the objects they contaminate *on contact.*

Many skin diseases are the result of poor hygienic practices. This is certainly true of athlete's foot, which is usually contracted in locker room facilities. The majority of athletes fail to carefully cleanse and dry their feet. When the feet are continually soaked with moisture plus microbes, infection is likely to occur. This could be remedied in part by adding tea tree oil to the janitorial cleansing solutions and by rubbing the pure oil on the feet and between the toes after showering. Bacterial skin infections, such as impetigo, boils and paronychia, may also be a consequence of poor hygiene. Impetigo occurs most frequently in children, who are notorious for failing to properly clean themselves. Tea tree oil is an excellent treatment for these conditions and may, in fact, be regarded as the *treatment of choice*.

The Environment

America is a land burdened by chemical toxicity. Since the turn of the century, thousands of synthetic chemicals have been produced. These chemicals, which are now distributed throughout the biosphere, were previously unknown to the universe. They are environmental anomalies and are precipitating the destruction of the universe as we know it. The loss of the ozone layer is just one example of the havoc they are wreaking.

Synthetic chemicals have caused widespread pollution of the soil, air and water. As a result there is no pure water, air or soil left in the world today.

The term "chemical" itself is largely misunderstood. The world and everything within it is made up of chemicals. Water is a chemical. A piece of bread consists of thousands of different chemicals.

Chemicals may be natural or synthetic. There are valuable synthetic chemicals, but most are harmful.

There is some overlap between the natural and synthetic. For instance, vitamin C is found naturally in certain foods such as tomatoes, citrus fruits and fresh vegetables. Vitamin C can also be produced synthetically. The typical vitamin C supplement, ascorbic acid, is an example of the synthetic form of this vitamin. All vitamin C supplements currently on the market are synthetic. Yet, researchers as well as those who use the vitamin known it has measurable biological effects. In this instance, the natural and synthetic are essentially the same.

Chemists attempts to duplicate nature are not always so successful. An excellent example is vitamin E. This vitamin is found naturally in many foods. Vitamin E is also produced synthetically. While the natural and synthetic are similar in structure, natural vitamin E is nearly three times more potent in terms of biological activity. This is an example of man's inability to mimic the powers of Nature.

Cyanide is an example of a highly lethal synthetic chemical. The botulism toxin, which is an entirely natural substance, is the most toxic chemical known, being lethal to humans and all other creatures in infinitesimal amounts. Aflatoxin, a natural chemical produced by certain molds, is the most powerful carcinogen ever to be tested. Even so, there are an infinitely greater number of synthetic toxic chemicals which are polluting the environment---and our bodies---than natural ones.

The distinction is incomparable. Natural chemicals degrade into harmless substances and will not pollute the environment. The majority of synthetic chemicals take years, if not decades, to decay. Some never decay.

Over the last 50 years there has occurred a massive growth in industries which produce various cleaning chemicals: soaps, detergents, solvents and germicides. While many of these agents are effective at cleaning filth and killing microbes, nearly all pollute the environment, causing irreparable damage to the soil, water and air. This emphasizes yet another attribute of tea tree oil. It is just as powerful as many commercial germicides but is safe for the environment. It is completely biodegradable. The worst environmental damage that it can cause is that it might kill a few microbes. It is likely that Nature can withstand that kind of toxicity.

Conclusion

The American public is interested in using natural remedies for the treatment of human ailments. Hundreds of thousands of Americans regard themselves as naturalists, taking little or no medication, that is unless it is "all-natural." Business experts are finding a universal theme among Americans: the interest in environmentally safe productions. Analysts have determined that as many as 90% of those interviewed would rather purchase environmentally safe products, and many of these consumers would be willing to pay extra for such products. This attitude is most pronounced in the area of personal health and hygiene because, while there is a general concern about polluting the environment, people are most concerned about avoiding the pollution of their own bodies.

Today's plague is degenerative disease. This categorization includes heart disease, diabetes, atherosclerosis Alzheimer's disease, arthritis and cancer. However, infectious diseases, particularly those transmitted through sexual contact, are rapidly infringing upon degenerative diseases as major killers. Plus, infectious diseases cause a significant amount of morbidity, i.e. the loss of quality of life.

In a sense America is a "sick" society. It is a society burdened by degenerative disease, toxic chemical exposure, nuclear radiation toxicity, junk food "toxicity" and drug abuse. However, many Americans do care about their health and would make every effort possible to preserve and enhance it.

Ironically, in spite of this pervasive environmental toxicity, the medical profession continues its emphasis on the use of drug therapy for the treatment of disease. In many diseases, drugs are the sole treatment offered. Americans are surrounded by enough poisons as it is and don't need to add to their toxic burdens. People wish to avoid making themselves more ill than they already are. The majority are willing and actually prefer to utilize non-toxic therapies, especially if their druggists and doctors recommend them.

The proof for tea tree oil's efficacy in the treatment of disease is just as strong as that for comparable over the counter or prescription medicines. In some instances the proof is stronger. Dozens of research articles have documented the tremendous utility, as well as safety, of tea tree oil in the treatment of disease. There should be no hesitation by medical professionals to recommend it.

There are numerous tea tree oil products currently on the market. Among those most useful are tea tree oil mouthwashes, antiseptic creams, shampoos, soaps, suppositories and, of course, the pure oil itself.

People wish to purchase products that achieve measurable results. Tea tree oil is a results producer and it does so in a wide range of conditions. That is why people will refill their stock of this versatile and valuable oil again and again. Tea tree oil should be in everyone's medicine cabinet.*

---

* Quality tea tree oil products may be difficult to procure. They can be purchased in some health food stores and a few pharmacies. Additionally, tea tree oil products, including tea tree oil, mouthwash, soap, animal shampoo, suppositories, toothpicks and lotion may be purchased via mail-order by calling (800) 243-5242. This number is for orders only, the minimum order being $30.00.

Conditions for which Tea Tree Oil has been Proven Useful
(Listed by Body Region)

Head and Neck

Dandruff
Seborrhea
Psoriasis
Eczema
Ringworm
Furunculosis
Razor cuts
Mastoiditis
Head lice
Cradle cap

Face

Razor cuts
Acne

Mouth, Throat and Ears

Canker sores
Cold sores
Pyorrhea
Cavities
Toothaches
Outer ear infections
Middle Ear infections
Sore throats
Colds
Thrush
Halitosis

Hands and Fingers

Paronychia
Fingernail fungus

Joints

Arthritis
Gout

Respiratory System

Bronchitis
Sinusitis
Croup
Tonsillitis

Urinary Tract

Cystitis

Rectum

Hemorrhoids
Rectal fissures

Genitals

Genital herpes
Genital warts
Vaginitis
Penile discharge
Excessive odor
Jock itch

Feet

Bromhidrosis
Toenail fungus
Ingrown Toenail
Calluses
Corns

Skin

Eczema
Psoriasis
Ringworm
Boils
Cuts
Abrasions
Scrapes
Puncture wounds
Bed sores
Varicose ulcers
Surgical incisions
Burns
Itchy skin
Scabies
Pilonidal cysts
Impetigo
Dermatitis
Allergic rashes, including poison ivy, oak and sumac
Animal bites, including those by dogs, humans, cats and snakes
Insect bites

List of Tea Tree Oil Products Currently Available

Pure tea tree oil
Antiseptic creams and ointments
Mouthwashes
Toothpicks
Germicides
Shampoos
Conditioner
Hand creams
Bar Soaps
Pet shampoos
Suppositories
Lozenges
Dental floss
Massage oil
Deodorant

Bibliography

Belew, P.W., Rosenberg, E.W., and B.R. Jennings. 1980. Activation of the alternative pathway of complement by Malessezia ovalis. *Mycopathologia* 70:187.

Duffy, J., Shoen, R.T., and L.H. Segal. 1991. Update on Lyme disease. *Patient Care* June 14, pp. 24-30.

Dzink, J.L., et al. 1985. Gram negative species associated with active destruction of periodontal lesions. *Clin. Periodontal.* 12:648-59.

Ferrari, F.A., et al. 1980. Inhibition of candidacidal activity of human neutrophil leukocytes by aminoglycoside antibiotics. *Antimicrob. Agents Chemo.* 17:87.

Foreman, A., and C.B. Smith. 1990. Vaginitis: systematically solving a bothersome problem. *Postgraduate Medicine* 88:123-32.

Goldman, H.M. 1986. Periodontal disease. III. Bacterial plaque as the primary etiological factor in periodontal disease. *Compend. Contin. Educ. Dent.* 7:198-205.

Goldman, H.M. 1986. Periodontal disease. IV. Calculus and other etiologic factors. *Ibid*, pp. 270-78.

Humphrey, M.E. 1930. A new Australian germicide. *Med. J. Aust.* 1:417.

Krause, W., Amathe Matheis, H., and K. Wulf. 1969. Fungaemia and funguria after oral administration of Candida albicans. *The Lancet* Mar. 22.

Martin, M.V., et al. 1984. An investigation of the role of true hypha production in the pathogenesis of experimental oral candidosis. *Sabouraudia J. Med. Vet. Mycolog.* 22:471.

Maruzzella, J.L., and L. Ligouri. 1958. The in vitro antifungal activity of essential oils. *J. Amer. Pharm. Assoc.* 47:250-4.

Medoff, G., and G.S. Kobayashi. 1991. Systemic fungal infections: an overview. *Hospital Practice* Feb. 15, pp. 41-52.

Noah, P.W. 1990. The role of microorganisms in psoriasis. *Seminars in Dermatology* 9:269-76.

Owens, R.C. 1981. Candidiasis: colonization and infection in the allergic patient. *Allergy Problems: Current Therapy Medical Education,* pp. 143-55.

Pena, E. 1962. Melaleuca alternifolia oil: its use for trichomonal vaginitis and other vaginal infections. *Obstetrics and Gynecology* 19:793-5.

Penfold, A., and R. Grant. 1923. The germicidal values of principle commercial eucalyptus oils and their pure constituents with observations on the values of concentrated disinfectants. *J. Proc. Royal Soc.* 57:80-89.

Penfold, A., and R. Grant. 1925. The germicidal values of some Australian essential oils and their pure constituents. Part III. *J. Proc. Royal Soc.* 59:346-50.

Penfold, A. 1937. Some notes on the essential oil of Melaleuca alternifolia. *Aust. J. Pharm.* Mar., p. 274.

Piccolella, E., et al. 1981. Generation of suppressor cells in the response of human lymphocytes to a polysaccharide from Candida albicans. *J. Immunol.* 126:2151.

Rivas, V.B., and T.J. Rogers. 1983. Studies on the cellular nature of Candida albicans induced suppression. *J. Immunol.* 130:376.

Rosenberg, W.E., Belew, P., and G. Bale. 1980. Effect of topical applications of heavy suspensions of killed Malassezia ovalis on rabbit skin. *Mycopathologia* 72:147-54.

Sanders, P.C., et al. 1986. The effects of a simplified mechanical oral hygiene regimen plus supragingival irrigation with chlorhexidine or metronidazole on subgingival plaque. *J. Clin. Periodont.* 13:237.

Seeling, M.S. 1966. Role of antibiotics in the pathogenesis of Candida infections. *Amer. J. Med.* 40:887.

Skinner, R.B., et al. 1985. Double-blind treatment of seborrheic dermatitis with 2% ketoconazole cream. *J. Amer. Acad. Dermatol.* 12:852.

Stobo, J.D., et al. 1976. Suppressor thymus-derived lymphocytes in fungal infection. *J. Clin. Investig.* 57:319.

Swerling, M.H., Owens, K.N., and R. Ruth. 1984. "Think Yeast"----the expanding spectrum of candidiasis. *J. South Carolina Med. Assoc.* 80:454-56.

Swords, G., and G.L.K. Hunter. 1978. Composition of Australian tea tree oil. *J. Agri. Food Chem.* 26:734-37.

Truss, C.O. 1978. Tissue injury induced by Candida albicans: mental and neurological manifestation. *J. Orthomol. Psych.* 7:17-35.

Truss, C.O. 1981. The role of Candida albicans in human illness. *J. Orthomol. Psych.* 10:228-38.

Umenai, T. 1978. Systemic candidiasis produced by oral Candida administration in mice. *Tohoku. J. Exp. Med.* 126:173.

van Palenstein Helderman, W.H. 1981. Microbial etiology of periodontal disease. *J. Clin. Periodontal.* 8:261.

Walker, M. 1972. Clinical investigation of Australian Melaluca alternifolia oil for a variety of common foot problems. *Current Podiatry*, April.

Walsh, L.J., and J. Longstaff. 1987. The antimicrobial effects of an essential oil on selected oral pathogens. *Periodontology* 8:11-15.

Witkin, S.S., et al. 1985. Inhibition of Candida albicans-induced proliferation by lymphocytes and sera from women with recurrent vaginitis. *Am. J. Obstet. Gynecol.* 147:809.

INDEX